W9-CDS-237

34-6

Acupuncture Therapy

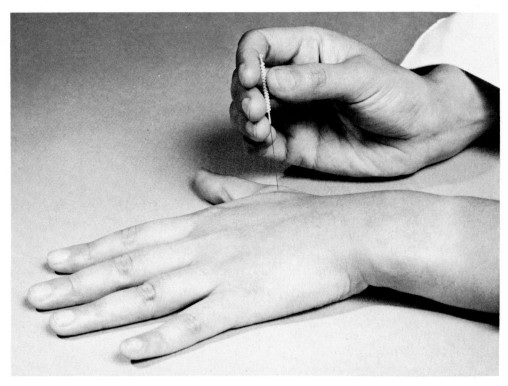

Temple University Press   *Philadelphia*

Acupuncture Therapy

Current Chinese Practice

Leong T. Tan
Margaret Y.-C. Tan
Ilza Veith

Foreword by Walter R. Tkach, M.D.

RM184. T325 1973

Temple University Press, Philadelphia 19122
© 1973 by Temple University. All rights reserved
Published 1973
Printed in the United States of America

International Standard Book Number: 0–87722–025–5
Library of Congress Catalog Card Number: 72–96004

LEONG T. TAN, M.D., F.A.C.S., is a practicing
urologist in San Francisco. MARGARET Y.-C.
TAN, M.S., Associate Specialist in the Department
of Medicine at the University of California San
Francisco, is a trained acupuncturist. ILZA VEITH,
M.A., Ph.D., is Professor and Vice Chairman of
the Department of Health Sciences at the University
of California San Francisco and a leading authority
on oriental medicine. She has written many books
and articles and is the translator of *The Yellow
Emperor's Classic of Internal Medicine.*

Second printing 1974

TO HANS
A Man for All Seasons

928963
EDUCATION

CONTENTS

FOREWORD

The recent resurgence of interest in acupuncture therapy may very well be due to President Richard Nixon's journey to the People's Republic of China. It has also been due to articles published by Dr. E. Grey Dimond and Dr. Paul Dudley White. The most scholarly presentation was made by Dr. Dimond in his articles in the *Journal of the American Medical Association.*

After we had visited the Friendship Hospital in Peking, I immediately reported to the President and related to him the operative procedures that we had observed. He was intensely interested, and the request was made that I review my notes and write a summary that would be of interest in America. This was done in articles in *Today's Health* and another widely disseminated journal. The happy surprise was the great number of physicians as well as members of the general public who wrote and asked for more information and about the possibility of visiting China to study the acupuncture procedure as it was used in anesthesia and for the relief of pain. Literally thousands of letters were received.

Three surgical procedures were observed, and when the value of the new anesthetic technique was realized, it was obvious that the medical profession outside of China could very well utilize this method. It is not a perfect anesthetic procedure, but the benefits derived from it were certainly impressive. As I thought about acupuncture-anesthesia in the months following, I realized that this was not anesthesia in the sense that we would describe it. I suggested to Dr. Ilza Veith that a new word should be coined. She suggested acupuncture-analgesia, but as we come to know more about it, I would hope that a more fitting and descriptive term will be found.

In the eight days that we spent in the People's Republic of China this new modality was discussed many times with the Chinese physicians. It was obvious that it had its finest application in the relief of pain. They made no extravagant claims as to cures for cancer, heart disease, and other illnesses that befall mankind. It appeared that they knew exactly at that time what they had and what they could do with it. It is my hope that in the near future we will be able to send a team to the People's Republic of China to study this procedure in detail in order to become proficient and to teach American physicians the value of acupuncture therapy and particularly its application to anesthesia.

Doctors Leong T. Tan and Ilza Veith and Mrs. Margaret Y.-C. Tan have written an excellent text and assembled what is probably our total knowledge of acupuncture outside of the People's Republic of China.

WALTER R. TKACH, M.D.

The White House

PREFACE

Until recently, a monograph on acupuncture would have attracted little or no interest in the Western world, much less in the United States. Acupuncture, it appeared, was a phenomenon that belonged to the realm of folklore, fantasy, mysticism, and indeed, even witchcraft. "A lot of hocus pocus" seemed to be the prevailing comment. In reality, however, acupuncture is a traditional mode of medical treatment in China, the practice of which has existed for thousands of years. Millions of patients, from personal experiences, can attest to the effect of needles, properly inserted at specific locations of the body: the palliation of certain afflictions, the alleviation of pain, and in recent years, the medical wonder of acupuncture-anesthesia or acupuncture-analgesia. As a simple, efficient, and, more important, effective means of medical therapy, acupuncture has successfully withstood the test of time, of scrutiny, and of acceptance. To those who remain skeptical of, or are baffled by, its accomplishments, this ancient art of healing deserves serious, responsible, and objective evaluation of its merits.

Many books have been written on this subject, both in Oriental and in Western languages. Judging from comments made by prospective students of this mode of therapy as well as from personal investigation of available literature, the authors found wanting an adequate source of instruction on the practical aspects of acupuncture treatment in the Western texts, specifically in the English language. It was to fill this particular void that the authors embarked on the preparation of this book. To this end, several current Chinese texts on acupuncture have been reviewed in detail and selectively translated. Information so gained forms the contents of this book.

As a medical procedure, the insertion and manipulation of acupuncture needles is fairly simple. For all practical purposes, no hazard to the general health of the patient is incurred provided, of course, that acupuncture is correctly practiced. On the strength of its simplicity and effectiveness, acupuncture has enjoyed a wide acceptance as a home cure performed by self-taught friends and family members. The problem that arises, however, is that acupuncture is by no means a cure-all. Serious pathological conditions that will not yield to needle treatment may be overlooked and remain undiagnosed by a medically untrained operator. A professional diagnosis is therefore at least as important for acupuncture therapy as it is for any other kind of medical intervention.

The present reception of acupuncture in Western, especially in American, scientific society raises memories of previous medical innovations, such as vaccination, anesthesia, antisepsis, chemotherapy, insulin, and antibiotics, to name just a few. Opinion of these innovations often gyrated between "myth" and "miracle." All were hotly debated, but it was a prominent American surgeon, John Collins Warren, who exclaimed after his first operation with ether anesthesia in 1846: "Gentlemen, this is no humbug!" Time will tell whether or not acupuncture will enter our vocabulary of medical household words and be taken for granted as a therapeutic method along with so many others.

Leong T. Tan, M.D., F.A.C.S.
Margaret Y.-C. Tan, M.S.
Ilza Veith, M.A., PH.D.

Acupuncture Therapy

INTRODUCTION

AMERICAN "DISCOVERY" OF ACUPUNCTURE

No aspect of the American rapprochement with China, including President Nixon's historic visit in February 1972, has caught the interest of the American public as much as have news items—quite incidental indeed—about the medical experience of a distinguished American correspondent. By suffering an appendicitis and undergoing an appendectomy, James Reston of the *New York Times* "discovered" acupuncture, a "discovery" that was made anew by most subsequent American visitors to China in 1971–72, including the President.

In fact, some of those who discovered acupuncture in the year of rapprochement were not completely incorrect in regarding it as a new modality that was somehow associated with Chairman Mao. But only acupuncture-anesthesia is actually a new phenomenon, hardly more than ten years old, and almost unknown outside of China proper. This aspect of acupuncture, important as it is, is really an innovation upon an ancient method of treatment, for acupuncture as an analgesic and as therapy stems from the neolithic age and is therefore at least seven thousand years old. Proof for this surprising statement is the existence of acupuncture needles made of flint, used long before the discovery of metal.

It is interesting that of all Western nations, scarcely any but the United States would have reacted to the sight of acupuncture with as much amazement and surprise. In most countries of Europe, especially France, Germany, Austria, England, and Russia, acupuncture therapy has long been known and practiced by physicians without discrimination from their scientific medical colleagues. Except for Russia, which adopted acupuncture as late as 1959, the other European countries became acquainted with this Chinese practice in the seventeenth and eighteenth centuries, when their colonial, diplomatic, or religious representatives returned from the Far East and spoke highly of the therapeutic methods they had observed. Here it should be stressed that the original oriental application of acupuncture was for the alleviation of the pains of arthritis, gout, and gastro-intestinal disturbances.

It was probably just because of these specific applications that acupuncture found such an interested reception in Europe, for gout in particular was a major bane of the well-born, of scholars, and especially of the most prominent of the physicians. As medical records and statistics had not come into use in those centuries, we do not know how effective acupuncture was in actually bringing relief from these painful afflictions, nor do we have these answers today.

WHAT IS ACUPUNCTURE?

Before continuing the story of acupuncture in the West, a few words should be said about the actual value of, and the rationale for, this procedure.

As we said above, acupuncture is part of the ancient Chinese medical system reaching back into prehistoric times. Its earliest documentation may be found in a medical treatise which was written in the third or fourth century B.C., *The Yellow Emperor's Classic of Internal Medicine.* According to Webster, the word "acupuncture" is derived from the Latin word *acus,* the needle, and *punctura,* a pricking, and means "a puncturing of bodily tissue for the relief of pain." It is performed by inserting sharp needles of various lengths into one or several of hundreds of points located all over the body, including the head and the extremities. These needles are inserted to various depths, rotated, left in situ, or immediately withdrawn.

It is difficult to find the rationale for the introduction of this uncommon therapy. Even in *The Yellow Emperor's Classic of Internal Medicine,* no such explanation is given. At the time this work was written, acupuncture must have been such a well-known form of therapy that explanations of its origin were considered unnecessary. In the course of history, however, a number of legends have arisen which furnish spurious (or perhaps even valid) explanations. The one most frequently cited is that ancient Chinese warriors, after having been injured by arrows in a variety of places, noticed the disappearance of pains of long standing and hence figured out a cause-and-effect relationship between the arrow wound and the unexpected amelioration or cure of their pains. Rather than believing in events that can scarcely be documented, it seems wiser to search for a rationale in the medical philosophy of the ancient Far East. Thus, what seems more likely than the apocryphal warriors is the early observation of the analgesic effect of massage, which also originated in China, that is, the kneading of specific parts of the body to bring about general relaxation and alleviation of pain.

As long as we do not have a documented Chinese history of the discovery of acupuncture, it will be important to understand its application and curative effect in terms of the ancient oriental natural philosophy. It needs to be stressed that the rationale for acupuncture is totally unrelated to any Western reasons for inserting needles into the human body: acupuncture needles are not hollow and do not serve to convey any material into the body, nor are they used to withdraw any body fluid. Attempts to bring acupuncture within the framework of modern medical science have as yet not solved the enigma.

All traditional Chinese medicine is based on the concept that, in composition and function, man is a microcosmic image of the universe and subject to identical laws. From time immemorial the Chinese were awed by the immutable course of nature, which they thought to be guided by *Tao* 道 , the Way. Tao prevailed in the creation of the world out of a state of chaos; Tao causes the ever-recurring changes from day to night, from light to darkness, from life to death, and is present in the coexistence of good and evil, of male and female. The two forces through which Tao acts were named *Yin* 陰 and *Yang* 陽 ; Yin, the female element, possesses all the negative qualities, and Yang, the male element, all the positive qualities. Since Tao was thought to be a unitary principle, neither of its two components ever existed alone, and in an absolute state. Even in the male there was an admixture of the female element; and in the female an admixture of the male.

In the universe, the harmonious working of the dual forces Yin and Yang expressed itself in the waning and waxing of the moon, the rising and setting of the sun, the growing and ripening of the crops and countless other sequential natural phenomena. Droughts, floods, storms, tidal waves, earthquakes and other disasters of nature were thought to be the result of an imbalance of Yin and Yang. Similarly, in man and beast, health resulted from the balance of the Yin and the Yang, and all diseases were thought to be due to a dyscrasia of these forces.

In the physical body, both human and animal, the vital essence *ch'i* 氣 , consisting of a harmonious mixture of Yin and Yang, was believed to be conveyed through twelve pairs of main ducts, plus two trunk ducts, which run in the front and back midline of the body. In the Western world these ducts or channels have come to be known as "meridians." The meridians emerge at the surface of the body at a certain number of carefully designated and presumably sensitive places which subsequently became known as acupuncture points. These traditioanlly numbered 365, to correspond with the number of days in the solar year.

As a consequence of these beliefs, the Chinese did not recognize a variety of diseases. They saw only disease as such, brought about by one cause—the disequilibrium of Yin and Yang within the vital force

—which could affect different parts of the body. A similar relationship was thought to exist between the pulse and each of the internal organs. Each wrist was assumed to contain not one but six pulses and both wrists, that is, twelve pulses, had to be palpated by the physician. Since the twelve pairs of meridians conveying the Yin and Yang were held to have a direct connection with every organ and part of the body, it was logical to assume that these channels furnished the easiest access to the seat of the disturbance. In response to individual symptoms, specific points were chosen for each needling treatment. By inserting needles into one or several points and by leaving them in situ for a certain length of time, the equilibrium of Yin and Yang was expected to be restored, possibly by the escape of disharmonious combinations.

Each of these points was believed to be the direct exponent of a specific and possibly diseased organ within the body. Such a belief appears to demonstrate a complete and deliberate disregard for any knowledge of the structure and function of the human body, in favor of a theory which obviated a systematic study of anatomy. This disregard persisted because anatomical dissection was taboo among the ancient Chinese, whose veneration of the ancestral personality demanded the burial of an inviolate body, that is, a body untouched by the probing instruments of anatomical dissection, or even the knife of the surgeon. It was thus possible to assume the actual existence of twelve pairs of meridians as channels for the vital essence which transported the life force of man.

Belief in the existence of the meridians persisted even after the introduction of the study of anatomy and scientific medicine into China, and after it had become evident that the meridians and acupuncture points could not actually be demonstrated as discrete anatomical structures. Only very recently a Korean researcher, Kim Bong-han, claimed to have discovered and demonstrated the existence of additional meridians which he called the Bong-han points.

SCIENTIFIC THEORIES ON ACUPUNCTURE

Western medicine cannot help but speculate about the scientific secret of acupuncture, and several theories have been suggested to account for the uncanny success of the oriental procedure.

Lacking a knowledge of the nature and function of the central nervous system and of the brain, which was not considered one of the major organs of the body, the traditional Chinese practitioners of acupuncture had to work with the concepts inherent in their philosophical theories of man's bodily function. Divested from concepts of Yin and Yang and "vital essence," however, the idea of dermal representation of internal organs in the cerebral cortex is not as fanciful as it appears at first glance. The work of men of such scientific sophistication as Ramussen and Penfield showed twenty-five years ago that each area of the surface of the skin is represented by a corresponding area in the cerebral cortex. This correspondence between skin and cerebral cortex probably also accounts for the beneficial effect of massage.

While the Rasmussen-Penfield theory was not specifically intended to explain acupuncture but may well be applied to it, other investigators have concentrated upon finding a physiological explanation for acupuncture-analgesia.

As was to be expected, the arrival of modern Western scientific medicine in China reduced the importance of the disequilibrium of Yin and Yang as pathogenic factors and made it desirable to look for scientific reasons for the efficacy of acupuncture treatment. This is all the more the case since acupuncture has reached the Western world, and especially the United States. Most frequently quoted among these scientific reasons is the hypothesis of R. Melzack of McGill University and Patrick Wall of the University College in London, whose studies on the physiology of pain yielded the gate control theory. The so-called Melzack-Wall theory suggests that the pathway of pain to the brain is determined by a "gate control cell" in the substantia gelatinosa in the dorsal horn of the spinal cord.

Although a certain element of scientific speculation remains in this proposition, a connection with acupuncture was developed on the basis of the Melzack-Wall theory. According to reports of recent visitors to the People's Republic of China, Chinese investigators have been proceeding along this line of thought in considering the role of cortex, thalamus and hypothalamus without, however, arriving at demonstrable conclusions (personal communication). In the United States, two scientists in Michigan, Dr. Calvin H. Chen, a professor at Wayne State University and assistant medical superintendent at Northville State Hospital, and Dr. Pang L. Man of the same institution, have formulated a concept to establish the thalamus as a second gate and have hence termed their hypothesis the "two-gate control theory."

It is important also to note here that according to the latter theory acupuncture needles produce only a mild, fairly painless stimulation causing the gates to be closed, so that painful sensations cannot pass through.

Further speculations on this theory have appeared in an article by H. C. Tien.

In all probability none of the above mentioned theories on the neurophysiological mechanism of acupuncture is the last word in the explanation of the needle therapy, and it is entirely uncertain whether it will eventually be one or several investigators in the People's Republic of China or Western researchers who will succeed in finding the scientific basis for this mysterious operation. The immediate and perhaps somewhat simplistic response of many American physicians who are not themselves familiar with acupuncture has often been that it can simply be equated with hypnosis, i.e., suggestion. This "explanation" can hardly be considered the correct one, since acupuncture is effective in the treatment of infants and also of a great variety of animals. Neither infants nor animals have as yet been known to be susceptible to hypnosis. In fact, Tibetan and Mongolian nomads have for centuries succeeded in producing insensibility to pain in their horses for purposes of veterinary intervention with acupuncture.

Moreover, in modern pain research, the difference between psychogenic pain and somatogenic pain is considered to be increasingly less significant. It is difficult, if not impossible, to dissociate the mind from painful ailments. As far as psychosomatic aspects of acupuncture therapy are concerned, it stands to reason that Mao Tse-tung's personal interest in the resurgence and extension of acupuncture endows the Chinese patient with such complete confidence in the procedure that he is free even of pre-operative apprehension. So far as the treatment of emotional illness is concerned, acupuncture seems to be effective in the relief of a great many psychogenic dysfunctions, such as frigidity and impotence, obesity and anorexia nervosa, insomnia and excessive fatigue, asthma, and migraine.

Acupuncture research is also going forward in all the European countries where it has been practiced so far. It is interesting to note that precisely those European nations which represent the cradle of modern medical science have accepted acupuncture as one of the therapeutic modalities open to the medical profession. The same is true in Japan, where acupuncturist physicians practice side by side with their Western-trained colleagues. This is because, centuries ago, Chinese medicine, and with it acupuncture, has found its way into all Asian countries which were pervaded by Chinese culture: Korea, Taiwan—in fact, all of Southeast Asia—but chiefly Japan.

MOXIBUSTION

Moxibustion is another form of therapy which developed in China in conjunction with acupuncture. It is the application to the established acupuncture points of small combustible cones of dried leaves of *Artemisia vulgaris,* or wormwood, which are ignited and burned down to the skin until a blister forms. Like acupuncture, moxibustion is also intended to restore homeostasis to the body. It was enthusiastically received in Japan, where it has continued to be practiced in its original form as an alternative to acupuncture, regardless of the burn scars that result. (The word "moxa" is derived from the Japanese *mogusa* "burning herb.") In China, on the other hand, moxibustion has continued in a somewhat attenuated form. Instead of bringing the burning moxa stick so close to the skin that a blister results, the moxa has been removed from the skin and is now used almost exclusively for heating the needles or warming the acupuncture point from a distance.

PRACTICAL APPLICATION

The sudden flurry of interest in the United States in the practice of acupuncture has caused many desperately ill patients to seek this apparent cure-all. In this they were disappointed, as there are very few physicians in the United States who are skilled acupuncturists. With the increasing demand for this method of treatment, however, many American physicians have evinced an interest in the actual techniques of acupuncture, which have so far been the domain of anonymous practitioners within the Chinese communities in this country. The few licensed physicians skilled in acupuncture usually have had full-time obligations in other fields of medicine, and practiced acupuncture as a "side-line" only. The many textbooks on acupuncture which have been published in France, Germany, Japan, and China are generally inaccessible to American readers. But quite apart from the linguistic or cultural differences that separate the American reader from the European and Oriental publications, it should be stressed that these are largely based upon the ancient traditional methods of acupuncture. In the People's Republic of China acupuncture therapy has undergone some refinement. From among the many hundreds of traditional acupuncture points those have been chosen which have come to be known as most effective in pain therapy and anesthesia. In addition to narrowing down and refining the number of ancient points, the Chinese have added new points which are not hallowed by tradition but which have yielded unexpectedly favorable results.

A number of these points also come into play in acupunctural "anesthesia," and it is this facet of acupuncture that has most deeply impressed Western medical observers on their visits to the People's Republic of China. Strictly speaking, the expression "acupuncture-anesthesia," though widely used, is somewhat of a misnomer. The proper nomenclature should probably be acupuncture-analgesia. Since no paralysis of the nerve centers with consequent muscle relaxation, loss of consciousness and of all sensations occurs as in inhalation anesthesia, the patient remains fully conscious and aware that he is being operated upon. However, he does not feel the pain or discomfort that would ordinarily be felt in surgery. Acupuncture preparatory to and during the operation results in analgesia in the surgical field sufficient to produce this effect with great safety.

Chapter 4 of this volume deals with acupuncture-anesthesia and demonstrates that its application must be based upon a sound general knowledge of, and accomplished skill in, acupuncture. The study of surgery would be unthinkable and the results disastrous without a solid foundation in anatomy, physiology and other basic disciplines. Similarly precarious would be the attempt to go into acupuncture-anesthesia without a thorough understanding and adequate skill in the entire field of acupuncture, qualifications which cannot be acquired in a quick "crash course." They demand extensive instruction, as the Chinese acupuncturists receive it, men or women, scientific physicians or "barefoot doctors."

For these reasons the authors of this book decided to base their work on selective translations from several modern books on acupuncture therapy, as it is currently used in the People's Republic of China.

LEGISLATIVE ACTION

In supplying this information the authors also have taken into consideration the twofold void that exists in America with regard to this method of therapy: the almost total lack of licensed medical personnel adequately trained in acupuncture, and—a consequence of the first—

the dearth of approved training and research facilities in this field. The whole matter has become a public concern, and it is noteworthy that recently the California State Legislature and the Governor have shown a remarkable understanding of this situation by promulgating, in August 1972, Assembly Bill No. 1500. This bill declares the performance of acupuncture by an unlicensed person not in violation of the Professional Code, when carried on in an approved medical school under the supervision of a licensed physician for the primary purpose of scientific investigation. Although the bill does not legalize the unlicensed healer to engage in private practice, it opens the way to draw on the skills of the traditional Chinese practitioner for legitimate research and aims at the eventual development of a force of licensed physicians in the United States trained in the practice of acupuncture.

Only three months later the California Legislature followed up Assembly Bill 1500 with the Duffy-Song Acupuncture Act, Assembly Bill No. 976. This act authorizes the performance of acupuncture by an unlicensed person, alone or in conjunction with other forms of traditional Chinese medicine, however imposing, at the same time the following conditions: a) All such techniques and procedures are performed under the direct supervision and diagnosis of a licensed physician and surgeon or, in the field of dentistry or oral surgery, of a licensed dentist, all of whom are required to be of unquestioned professional standing. b) The supervising licensee submits, prior to commencing such supervision, a report to the Board of Medical Examiners containing his or her own name and address and the name and address of the unlicensed performers, together with a description of the project investigating acupuncture. The act designates the scientific investigation of acupuncture as its primary purpose and recognizes that the recent rising interest in acupuncture and other forms of traditional Chinese medicine has stimulated a desire on the part of practitioners of modern Western medicine to explore the aforementioned disciplines. The sponsors of this legislation seemed to feel that the medical profession—if it so elects—would be in a position to conclude preparations for the full practice of acupuncture within a reasonable span of time. Therefore the provisions of the Duffy-Song Act were to be operative only until December 31, 1975. The Duffy-Song Acupuncture Act, however, was vetoed by the Governor of California, in January 1973, with this comment: "The research effort at Medical Schools is now under way. Until further research has been completed, a broadening of authority to practice acupuncture is premature. The State Board of Medical Examiners has requested that the bill be vetoed. I concur in their opposition at this time."

It now remains to be seen whether the American medical world can integrate a therapeutic procedure which, for the time being, seems to lie beyond a scientific rationale. The fact persists, however, that acupuncture has proven effective to untold hundreds of millions of sufferers for thousands of years of healing practice.

THE ESSENTIALS
OF ACUPUNCTURE

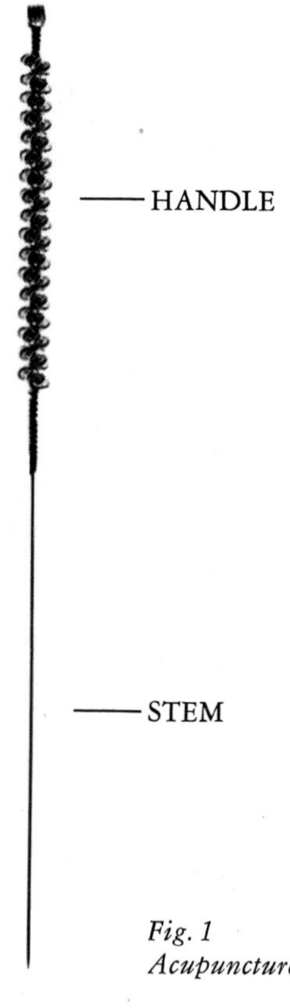

————HANDLE

————STEM

Fig. 1
Acupuncture needle

1   THE ESSENTIALS
OF ACUPUNCTURE

The practice of acupuncture depends on acquaintance with the following features: acupuncture needles, techniques of acupuncture, moxibustion, electric acupuncture, and identification of acupuncture points. The practitioner must be familiar with the insertion of needles, the directions of needle insertion, responses to needle insertion, and methods of treatment.

ACUPUNCTURE NEEDLES

The two parts of a needle are its handle and its stem. The handle is made of either copper or aluminum while the stem is nowadays manufactured from stainless steel. The needles vary in length from 0.5 inches to 4.0 inches. The selection of the appropriate needle is dictated by the location of the acupuncture point. Needles 0.5 inches long are usually used for head and facial points, while needles 1.5 to 2.0 inches long are used for points located on the torso, arms, and legs. Needles 3.0 to 4.0 inches long are reserved for points situated in deep tissue or thick musculature, such as the glutei muscles.

Acupuncture needles also vary in diameter, from 26 gauge (0.45 mm) to 32 gauge (0.28 mm). Most frequently used are 30 gauge needles; for points around the eyes, 32 gauge; and for situations in which strong sensory stimulation is desired or for puncturing the skin to produce a drop of blood (blood-letting), 26 to 28 gauge.

TECHNIQUES OF ACUPUNCTURE

Insertion of needle. Preparation prior to acupuncture includes scrubbing the hands, prepping the site of insertion with alcohol, and examining the sterile needle for any defect. The two most popular techniques for inserting the needle are the following (see Fig. 2).

1. Using either the index finger or thumb of the left hand, digital pressure is applied to the site immediately adjacent to the acupuncture point. The handle of the needle is held between the thumb and index finger of the right hand while the third and fourth fingers support the stem. The needle is then directed towards the acupuncture point. By applying gentle pressure and continuously twirling the handle of the needle simultaneously, the needle is inserted through the skin at the acupuncture point to the depth desired.

2. An alternative technique, which is preferred for inserting needles of 3.0 inches or longer, is the following: holding the distal end of the needle between the thumb and index finger of the right hand, apply digital pressure to the site immediately adjacent to the acupuncture point with the left thumb or index finger, and then, with a jab, insert the needle through the skin at the acupuncture point. Next, after changing hands to support the stem of the needle with the left index finger and thumb, the needle is advanced to the proper depth by applying pressure and continuously twirling its handle with the index finger and thumb of the right hand.

Certain maneuvers may facilitate needle insertion when the following anatomical features are encountered. At locations where little musculature is present, one may pick up the skin and subcutaneous tissue with the fingers of the left hand for inserting the needle (Fig. 2). In addition, skin that hangs loosely or is wrinkled is stretched taut before inserting the needle into it.

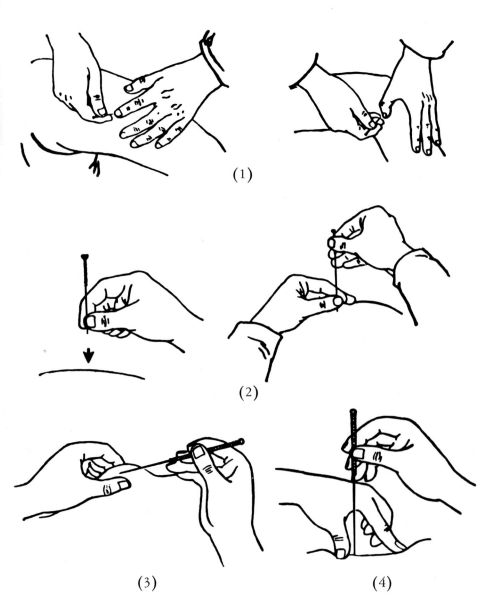

Fig. 2
Techniques of needle insertion

Directions of needle insertion (Fig. 3). Accurate insertion of the needle, with reference to direction, angle, and depth, must be achieved in order to produce safe and effective results. The directions and angles of insertion are as follows:

1. Perpendicular insertion. The needle and the skin at the acupuncture point should form an angle of approximately 90 degrees. This angle of insertion is generally used for deep insertion of the needle.
2. Diagonal insertion. The needle and the skin form an angle of between 30 and 60 degrees. This angle is also mostly used for deep insertion.
3. Horizontal insertion. The needle and the skin should form an angle of between 10 and 20 degrees. This is the usual angle of insertion at locations with minimal subcutaneous tissue or musculature.

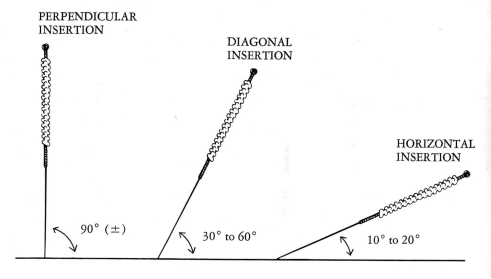

PERPENDICULAR
INSERTION

DIAGONAL
INSERTION

HORIZONTAL
INSERTION

90° (±)   30° to 60°   10° to 20°

Fig. 3
Directions of needle insertion

The depth to which a needle is to be inserted is singular to each acupuncture point and is described in chapter 2. In general, a sensory response will be evoked from the patient when the needle reaches the appropriate depth.

Responses to successful needle insertions. Acupuncture, successfully executed, will elicit a variety of sensory responses from the patient. These range from a feeling of numbness at the acupuncture point to a sense of heaviness, dull ache, or tingling sensation which may be localized or radiating. These responses are known in Chinese as *Te-ch'i* 得氣 ("acquiring vital energy"). Puncturing of points on the head or face generally furnishes a sensation of heaviness or fullness; points located in deep musculature, numbness or a tingling sensation; while puncturing points at the fingertips usually produces a painful sensation.

Methods of treatment. The following methods are usually employed.

1. Short course therapy. Following correct positioning of the needle, as evidenced by appropriate sensory response from the patient, the needle is continuously twirled or agitated rapidly with an up-and-down motion for 10 to 20 seconds and then removed.
2. Intermittent therapy. The needle is twirled for several seconds intermittently with rest periods of a few minutes in between.
3. Continuous therapy. The needle is continuously twirled for several minutes or hours, or until symptomatic relief is obtained.

At the conclusion of treatment, the needle is removed by applying counterpressure on the skin adjacent to the needle with the left index finger as the needle is withdrawn while slowly twirling it with the right index finger and thumb.

Course of therapy. In general, acute conditions may be treated one to three times a day. Chronic diseases, however, are treated once every one to three days for a total of 10 to 20 treatments. This constitutes one course of therapy and it may be repeated after a rest period of one to two weeks.

MOXIBUSTION

Moxibustion—the application of heat to acupuncture points by burning *ai* or moxa, the dried leaves of *Artemesia vulgaris*—is used by itself or to complement acupuncture in the treatment of diseases. Heat can be applied directly by burning small cones of moxa at specific acupuncture points or indirectly by (1) heating an inserted needle with an ignited moxa cigarette (moxa rolled up in tissue paper like a cigarette), (2) holding the moxa cigarette approximately 0.5 inches above the acupuncture point when a needle is not used, or (3) heating a small pile of moxa on a slice of ginger placed over the acupuncture point. Treatment may be carried out for 10 to 20 minutes. Moxibustion is not recommended for facial points, superficial points that are in close vicinity to blood vessels, and points on the abdomen and back of pregnant women. It is, however, most effective in relieving arthralgias and abdominal pain.

ELECTRIC ACUPUNCTURE

A modality of recent origin, the utilization of an electric current for stimulation of an inserted needle is now widely and routinely employed in the practice of acupuncture. This innovation provides the following advantages:

1. It effectively replaces stimulation by manual twirling which can be quite fatiguing when treatment is prolonged.
2. The degree of stimulation can be accurately and evenly adjusted.
3. A stronger degree of stimulation can be achieved than by manual twirling.

Technique. Two acupuncture points must be used, one for each of the electrical leads. Following successful insertion of the needles, as evidenced by the proper sensory response, each needle is connected to one of the leads which in turn are attached to a direct current 9-volt battery power unit. The power unit is then turned on and the electric

current slowly increased. As with manual twirling, a variety of responses such as paresthesia, numbness, a sense of fullness or heaviness, or a mild degree of muscle spasm will be elicited when the optimum amount of electric stimulation is administered. During the course of treatment, the patient's threshold of tolerance to the stimulation usually increases. Consequently, his sensory responses will be diminished. When this occurs, it will be necessary to increase the electric output to reestablish an effective degree of stimulation. Continuously increasing the electric current, however, may not be desirable and can be avoided by continually varying the output of the current, thereby preventing the patient from developing a tolerance to the stimulation. As a rule, acupuncture points on the face and below the elbow and the knee are more sensitive to electric stimulation than are points located elsewhere on the body.

Electric acupuncture is usually applied for approximately 10 minutes but this duration may be extended to four or five hours without producing any known ill-effects. Caution, however, should be exercised when using this form of treatment on patients with severe cardiac diseases.

This mode of therapy is especially noted for its effectiveness in inducing analgesia and in the treatment of diseases of the nervous system.

POSSIBLE COMPLICATIONS OF ACUPUNCTURE
Complications from acupuncture, though infrequent, can nevertheless occur, especially when it is incorrectly practiced.

Asepsis in technique, properly observed, should eliminate the possibilities of infection and hepatitis. An ill-advised or inadvertent insertion of the needle into the peritoneal cavity with subsequent injury to the organs therein may theoretically cause peritonitis and/or hemoperitoneum, even though this rarely occurs in practice. Ecchymoses at sites of acupuncture are not uncommon. They are more often seen with acupuncture-anesthesia when the needles are usually stimulated continuously for long periods. The ecchymoses essentially are of no clinical significance. However, serious bleeding may ensue from inadvertent needling of vital organs or major blood vessels. Similarly, pneumothorax and hemothorax are potential hazards associated with acupuncture in the region of the thorax. The insertion of needles into the central nervous system is also to be avoided when performing acupuncture at points along the vertebral column as transient paralysis may result from strong stimulation of the central nervous system.

IDENTIFICATION OF ACUPUNCTURE POINTS

Hundreds of acupuncture points have been documented in the Chinese literature of various periods. The majority of these points are located in linear arrangement along the major "meridians" of the body, of which twelve major pairs plus two at the midline of the body, front and back, have been established by tradition. Thus, except for the points situated along the midline meridians, each acupuncture point is paired, its companion point being located in a mirror-image position.

During the course of an ailment, localized pain may be elicited by applying digital pressure on certain points of the body. These tender spots, which are known as "pressure points," are also used as acupuncture points. Although the locations of these pressure points are not specific, they are usually found in the vicinity of the affected areas, as in the case of muscle spasms. However, they may also be located at a site distant to the afflicted organ, as exemplified by the acupuncture point for the treatment of appendicitis, Lan-wei-hsüeh, and the point for the relief of biliary colic, Tan-nang-hsüeh.

In the identification of a specific acupuncture point, reliance is placed on two systems.

1. Body-inch method of measurement. One body-inch is equivalent to the distance between the joint creases of the interphalangeal joints of the patient's middle finger when it is flexed. It is also equivalent to the width of the patient's thumb. Furthermore, the

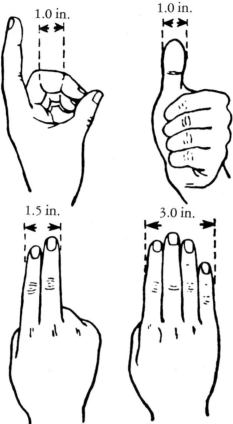

Fig. 4
Body-inch measurement

total width of the patient's four fingers (excluding the thumb) measures up to 3.0 body-inches, while the combined width of the index and middle fingers is equivalent to 1.5 body-inches (Fig. 4). In this text, all inches mentioned in reference to the location of an acupuncture point are body-inches, which are specific for each patient.

2. Conventional anatomical landmarks such as easily identifiable bony structures, muscles, tendons, and external features.

MOST COMMONLY USED
ACUPUNCTURE POINTS

2 MOST COMMONLY USED ACUPUNCTURE POINTS

The description of each acupuncture point covers its location in relation to conventional anatomical landmarks, indications for its use (diseases and symptoms amenable to treatment by stimulation of the acupuncture point in question), the recommended direction and depth of needle insertion, and a mention of moxa heating when its use will complement acupuncture. The last is not recommended when omitted in the text. When recommended, indirect heating is preferred.

The name of each acupuncture point is given in its transliterated version. In order to facilitate identification, an anatomical reference is ascribed to each point wherever possible, along with the organ specificity of the point. Each point is numbered within the section on points of that area of the body and the following abbreviations for the sections are used in cross-reference: HN for Head and Neck, UE for Upper Extremities, LE for Lower Extremities, CA for Chest and Abdomen, and B for Back. Thus, for example, HN–8 refers to Hsia-kuan, point 8 in the section on points of the head and neck.

POINTS OF THE HEAD AND NECK

1. Pê-hui, *vertex (Fig. 5)*

Location. At the vertex of the skull or at the point of intersection of a line joining the upper tips of the ears and a line drawn from the middle of the forehead directly towards the vertex.

Indications. Headaches, dizziness, syncope, hypertension, and rectal prolapse.
Technique. Horizontal insertion towards the front or the back of the skull to a depth of 0.5 to 1.0 inches.
Moxa heating. 5 to 20 minutes.

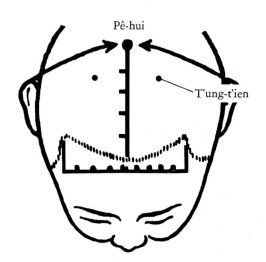

Fig. 5

2. T'ung-t'ien *(Fig. 5)*

Location. 1.5 inches lateral to a point 1.0 inches directly anterior to the point Pê-hui (HN–1).
Indications. Nasal infections (rhinitis, rhinorrhea), and headache.
Technique. Horizontal insertion anteriorly or posteriorly to a depth of 0.5 to 1.0 inches.
Moxa heating. 5 to 20 minutes.

3. T'ai-yang, *temporal (Fig. 6)*

Location. At the temple, at a point 1.0 inches directly posterior to the midpoint of a line joining the lateral canthus of the eye and the lateral margin of the eyebrow.

Indications. Temporal headaches, facial paralysis, tic douloureux, and eye diseases.

Technique. Perpendicular insertion 0.3 to 0.5 inches deep.

4. Yang-pê, *frontal (Fig. 7)*

Location. At a point one-third the distance of a line drawn directly upwards from the midpoint of the eyebrow to the hairline.

Indications. Facial paralysis, frontal headache, night blindness, and glaucoma.

Technique. Horizontal insertion laterally or medially 0.5 to 1.0 inches deep.

5. Shuai-ku, *supratemporal (Fig. 6)*

Location. 1.5 inches directly above the superior margin of the ear.

Indications. Temporal headache.

Technique. Horizontal insertion anteriorly to a depth of 0.5 to 1.0 inches.

Moxa heating. 3 to 5 minutes.

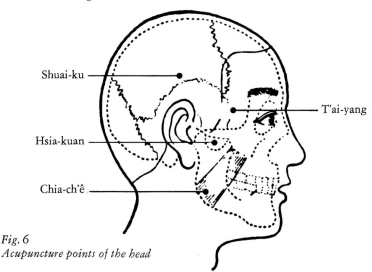

Fig. 6
Acupuncture points of the head

Fig. 7
Acupuncture points of the face

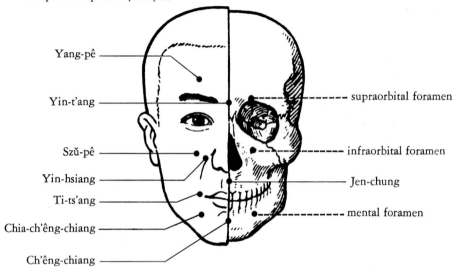

6. Yin-t'ang, *glabella (Fig. 7)*

   Location. At the glabella, midway between the medial margins of
   the eyebrows.
   Indications. Headache, dizziness, and nasal infections.
   Technique. Horizontal insertion, caudad, 0.5 to 1.0 inches deep.

7. Szŭ-pê, *infraorbital foramen (Fig. 7)*

   Location. At the infraorbital foramen or at a point one index finger's width directly inferior to the midpoint of the infraorbital
   margin.
   Indications. Facial paralysis, tic douloureux, nasal infections, and
   eye diseases.
   Technique. Perpendicular insertion 0.2 to 0.3 inches deep or horizontal insertion, caudad, 0.3 to 0.5 inches deep.

8. Hsia-kuan, *infratemporal fossa (Fig. 6)*

Location. In the infratemporal fossa, immediately anterior to the head of the mandible, or at a point one index finger's width anterior to the tragus of the ear. The head of the mandible can be easily palpated if the patient opens and closes the mouth.

Indications. Facial paralysis, tic douloureux, toothache, otitis media, and painful disorders of the mandibular joint.

Technique. Perpendicular insertion 0.3 to 1.5 inches deep, or diagonal insertion anteriorly or posteriorly to a depth of 0.5 to 0.8 inches, or horizontal insertion towards the corner of the mouth 1.5 inches deep.

9. Chia-ch'ê, *masseter (Fig. 6)*

Location. When the teeth are clenched, the point can be located in the body of the masseter muscle, one index finger's breadth anterior and superior to the angle of the mandible.

Indications. Toothache, facial paralysis, mumps, and spasm of the masseter muscle.

Technique. Perpendicular insertion 0.5 inches deep.

Moxa heating. 5 to 10 minutes.

10. Ching-ming, *medial canthus (Fig. 8)*

Location. With the eye closed, the point is 0.1 inches medial and slightly superior to the medial canthus of the eye.

Indications. Diseases of the eye.

Technique. Perpendicular insertion 0.2 to 0.6 inches deep. For treatment of myopia, the depth of insertion is 1.0 to 1.5 inches without any twirling of the needle.

11. Ch'êng-ch'i, *mid-infraorbital margin (Fig. 8)*

Location. Immediately superior to the midpoint of the infraorbital margin.

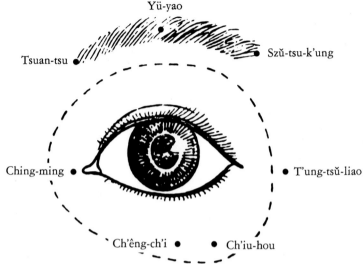

Fig. 8
Acupuncture points of the eye

Indications. Myopia and optic nerve disorders.
Technique. Perpendicular insertion 1.0 to 1.5 inches, with the patient looking upwards.

12. Ch'iu-hou *(Fig. 8)*

Location. Midpoint between the lateral border of the infraorbital margin and the point Chêng-ch'i (HN–11).
Indications. Optic nerve disorders, glaucoma, and myopia.
Technique. Perpendicular insertion 1.0 to 1.5 inches deep, with the patient looking upwards.

13. T'ung-tsŭ-liao, *lateral canthus (Fig. 8)*

Location. 0.5 inches directly lateral to the lateral canthus.
Indications. Diseases of the eye and headache.
Technique. Horizontal insertion posteriorly 0.5 to 1.0 inches deep.

34

14. Yü-yao, *mid-eyebrow (Fig. 8)*

> *Location.* At the midpoint of the eyebrow.
> *Indications.* Diseases of the eye.
> *Technique.* Horizontal insertion laterally or medially 0.5 to 1.0 inches deep.

15. Tsuan-tsu, *superciliary arch (Fig. 8)*

> *Location.* At the superciliary arch or medial margin of the eyebrow.
> *Indications.* Diseases of the eye and headache.
> *Technique.* Horizontal insertion, caudad, 0.3 to 0.5 inches deep, or perpendicular insertion 0.2 to 0.3 inches deep.

16. Szǔ-tsu-k'ung, *lateral eyebrow (Fig. 8)*

> *Location.* At the lateral margin of the eyebrow.
> *Indications.* Diseases of the eye and headache.
> *Technique.* Horizontal insertion posteriorly or medially 0.3 to 0.5 inches deep.

17. Yin-hsiang, *nasolabial fold (Fig. 7)*

> *Location.* At the superior aspect of the nasolabial fold.
> *Indications.* Nasal congestion, rhinitis, and facial paralysis.
> *Technique.* Horizontal insertion superiorly or caudad to a depth of 0.2 to 0.3 inches.

18. Jen-chung, *intermaxillary suture (Fig. 7)*

> *Location.* In the intermaxillary suture and at a point one-third of the distance from the anterior nasal spine to the midpoint of the upper lip.

Indications. Syncope, epilepsy, shock, painful disorders and swelling of the face, and excessive salivation in children.
Technique. Horizontal insertion, superiorly, 0.3 to 0.5 inches deep.

19. Ti-ts'ang *(Fig. 7)*

Location. One index finger's breadth directly lateral to the corner of the mouth.
Indications. Facial paralysis, tic douloureux, and excessive salivation.
Technique. Horizontal insertion 0.3 to 0.7 inches deep, towards the angle of the mandible.
Moxa heating. 3 to 10 minutes.

20. Ch'êng-chiang, *symphysis menti (Fig. 7)*

Location. One index finger's width inferior to the mucocutaneous line of the lower lip at the symphysis menti, or below the midpoint of the lower lip.
Indications. Facial paralysis, toothache, and gingivitis.
Technique. Horizonal insertion, laterally, 1.0 to 1.5 inches deep.

21. Chia-ch'êng-chiang, *mental foramen (Fig. 7)*

Location. 1.0 inches lateral to the point Ch'eng-chiang (HN–20), at the mental foramen.
Indications. Facial paralysis and tic douloureux.
Technique. Perpendicular insertion 0.2 to 0.3 inches deep.

22. Êrh-mên, *superior tragus (Fig. 9)*

Location. Immediately anterior to the superior margin of the tragus of the ear.
Indications. Deafness, tinnitus, and otitis media.

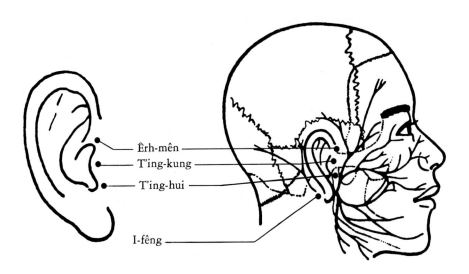

Êrh-mên

T'ing-kung

T'ing-hui

I-fêng

Fig. 9

Technique. With the patient's mouth open, perpendicular insertion 1.5 to 3.0 inches deep or diagonal insertion, caudad, to a depth of 2.0 to 3.0 inches.
Moxa heating. 3 to 5 minutes.

23. T'ing-kung, *mid-tragus (Fig. 9)*

Location. Immediately anterior to the middle portion of the tragus of the ear. Applying digital pressure on this point will occlude the external auditory meatus.
Indications. Deafness, tinnitus and otitis media.
Technique. With the patient's mouth open, perpendicular insertion to a depth of 0.3 to 1.5 inches.
Moxa heating. 3 to 5 minutes.

24. T'ing-hui, *inferior tragus (Fig. 9)*

Location. Immediately anterior to the inferior margin of the tragus of the ear.
Indications. Deafness, tinnitus, and otitis media.
Technique. With the patient's mouth open, perpendicular insertion, slightly posteriorly, to a depth of 1.0 to 2.0 inches.
Moxa heating. 3 to 5 minutes.

25. Fêng-ch'ih *(Fig. 10)*

Location. Midpoint of a line joining the tip of the mastoid process to the posterior midline, in the groove between the trapezius and sternocleidomastoideus.
Indications. Influenza, dizziness, headache, neck pain, hypertension, and tinnitus.
Technique. Diagonal insertion, medially and slightly caudad, 0.5 to 0.8 inches deep.
Moxa heating. 3 to 5 minutes.

26. Ya-mên, *C1–C2 (Fig. 10)*

Location. At the posterior midline, 0.5 inches above the hairline (between the first and second cervical vertebrae).
Indications. Mutism, deafness, occipital headache, torticollis, and mental disorders.
Technique. With the patient's head slightly flexed, perpendicular insertion, without any twirling motion, to a depth of approximately 1.0 inches. Successful penetration will elicit a localized sensation of pressure or fullness. However, should the patient experience paresthesia of all extremities, the needle should be immediately withdrawn.

27. T'ien-chu, *paravertebral C1–C2 (Fig. 10)*

Location. 1.5 inches lateral to the point for Ya-mên (HN–26) or

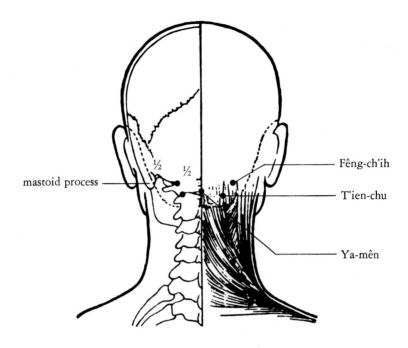

mastoid process ——

½ ½

—— Fêng-ch'ih

—— T'ien-chu

—— Ya-mên

Fig. 10

at the lateral border of the insertion of the trapezius.

Indications. Occipital headache and torticollis.

Technique. Perpendicular insertion approximately 0.5 inches deep.

Moxa heating. 5 minutes.

28. I-fêng, *post-auricular (Fig. 9)*

Location. In the groove between the ear lobe and the mastoid process.

Indications. Deafness, tinnitus, otitis media, facial paralysis, and mumps.

Technique. Perpendicular insertion, slightly caudad, 0.5 to 1.0 inches deep.

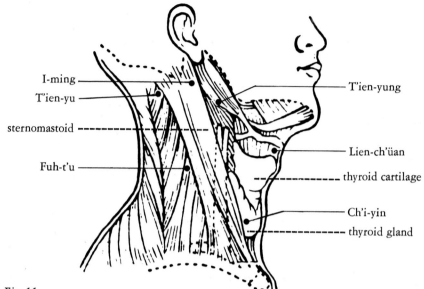

Fig. 11
Acupuncture points of the neck

29. I-ming, *mastoid process (Fig. 11)*

Location. Immediately below the tip of the mastoid process.
Indications. Tinnitus, myopia, optic nerve atrophy, cataracts, insomnia, mumps, and neurasthenia.
Technique. Perpendicular insertion 0.5 to 1.0 inches deep.

30. T'ien-yung, *mandibular angle (Fig. 11)*

Location. Immediately posterior and inferior to the angle of the mandible and anterior to the sternocleidomastoideus.
Indications. Tonsillitis, swelling and painful disorders of the neck.
Technique. Perpendicular insertion to a depth of 0.5 to 1.0 inches.
Moxa heating. 3 to 5 minutes.

31. T'ien-yu, *post-mastoid process (Fig. 11)*

Location. Immediately posterior and inferior to the mastoid process at the hairline or at the posterior margin of the insertion of the sternocleidomastoideus.
Indications. Tinnitus, deafness, torticollis, and pharyngitis.
Technique. Perpendicular insertion approximately 0.5 inches deep.
Moxa heating. 3 to 5 minutes.

32. Fuh-t'u, *mid-sternocleidomastoideus (Fig. 11)*

Location. 3.0 inches directly lateral to the laryngeal prominence of the thyroid cartilage at the posterolateral margin of the sterno-cleidomastoideus.
Indications. Hoarseness and dysphagia.
Technique. Perpendicular insertion to a depth of 0.3 to 0.5 inches.
Moxa heating. 5 to 10 minutes.

33. Lien-ch'üan, *supra laryngeal prominence (Fig. 11)*

Location. At the midline, immediately superior to the laryngeal prominence and inferior to the hyoid bone.
Indications. Numbness of the tongue, mutism, and dysarthria.
Technique. Perpendicular insertion approximately 0.5 inches deep.
Moxa heating. 3 to 5 minutes.

34. Ch'i-yin, *thyroid (Fig. 11)*

Location. In either lobe of the thyroid gland at the level of the cricoid cartilage.
Indications. Goiter.
Technique. Perpendicular insertion 0.5 to 1.5 inches deep towards the center of the lobe, but not beyond it.

Table 1

SUMMARY OF ACUPUNCTURE POINTS OF THE HEAD AND NECK

LOCATION		NAME	COMMON INDICATIONS	SPECIFIC INDICATIONS
	Vertex	Pê-hui, T'ung-t'ien	Vertical headache	Pê-hui: Rectal prolapse, diseases of the brain; T'ung-t'ien: Diseases of the nose
Head	Temporal	Shuai-ku, T'ai-yang	Diseases of head — Temporal headache	T'ai-yang: Eye disease, facial paralysis, tic douloureux
	Frontal	Yang-pê, Yin-t'ang	Frontal headache	Yang-pê: Eye diseases, facial paralysis; Yin-t'ang: Diseases of the brain and nose
Malar		Szŭ-pê, Chia-ch'ê, Hsia-kuan	Diseases of the trigeminal nerve and facial nerve	Szŭ-pê: Diseases of the eye and nose; Chia-ch'ê: Mumps, toothache; Hsia-kuan: Diseases of ear, toothache
Eye		Ching-ming, Ch'êng-ch'i, Ch'iu-hou, T'ung-tsŭ-liao, Tsuan-tsu, Yü-yao, Szŭ-tsu-k'ung	Eye diseases	T'ung-tsŭ-liao and Szŭ-tsu-k'ung: Temporal headache; Tsuan-tsu: Frontal headache

	Points	Diseases	Indications
Nose	Yin-hsiang		Yin-hsiang: Diseases of the nose, facial paralysis
Ear	Êrh-mên T'ing-kung T'ing-hui I-fêng	Ear diseases	I-fêng: Facial paralysis, mumps
Mouth	Jen-chung Ti-ts'ang Ch'êng-chiang Chia-ch'êng-chiang	Diseases of mouth and teeth	Jen-chung: Syncope, salivation Ti-ts'ang: Salivation, tic douloureux Chia-ch'êng-chiang: Tic douloureux
Neck — Back	Ya-mên Fêng-ch'ih T'ien-chu	Diseases of back of neck	Fêng-ch'ih: Hypertension, tinnitus, dizziness, influenza Ya-mên: Mutism
Neck — Side	I-ming T'ien-yung T'ien-yu	Diseases of side of neck	I-ming: Mumps, diseases of ear and eye, insomnia, neurasthenia T'ien-yung: Tonsillitis T'ien-yu: Diseases of ear and throat
Neck — Front	Fuh-t'u Lien-ch'üan Ch'i-yin	Diseases of front of neck	Fuh-t'u: Dysphagia and hoarseness Lien-ch'üan: Mutism, numbness of the tongue Chi-yin: Goiter

POINTS OF THE UPPER EXTREMITY

1. Chü-ku, *claviculo-scapular spine angle (Fig. 12)*

   Location. At the angle formed by the clavicle and the spine of the scapula.
   Indications. Painful disorders of the shoulder.
   Technique. Perpendicular insertion to a depth of 0.5 to 1.0 inches.
   Moxa heating. 5 to 10 minutes.

2. Chien-yü, *pre-acromion (Figs. 13 and 14)*

   Location. With the arm abducted to a horizontal position, the point is located in a small depression immediately anterior to the distal tip of the acromion.
   Indications. Painful disorders of the shoulder and upper arm, and paralysis of the upper extremity.

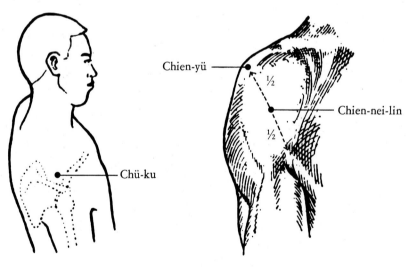

Fig. 12   Fig. 13

Technique. After identification of the point and with the arm in a dependent position, perpendicular insertion, in a direction approximately parallel to the clavicle to a depth of 0.5 to 1.0 inches.
Moxa heating. 5 to 15 minutes.

3. Chien-nei-lin, *supra anterior axillary fold (Fig. 13)*

Location. Midpoint of a line between the point Chien-yü (UE–2) and the anterior axillary fold.
Indications. Painful disorders of the shoulder and upper arm, and paralysis of the upper extremity.
Technique. Perpendicular insertion 1.0 to 1.5 inches deep.
Moxa heating. 5 to 20 minutes.

4. Chien-liao, *post-acromion (Fig. 14)*

Location. In the depression immediately posterior to the distal tip of the acromion (easier to identify when the arm is abducted to a horizontal position).
Indications. Painful disorders of the shoulder and upper arm, and paralysis of the upper extremity.
Technique. Perpendicular insertion towards the axilla to a depth of approximately 1.5 to 2.0 inches.
Moxa heating. 5 to 20 minutes.

5. Nao-yü, *infra scapular spine (Fig. 14)*

Location. In the fossa immediately below the spine of the scapula and directly above the posterior axillary fold.
Indications. Painful disorders of the shoulder and upper arm, and paralysis of the upper extremity.
Technique. Perpendicular insertion to a depth of 1.0 to 1.5 inches.
Moxa heating. 5 to 20 minutes.

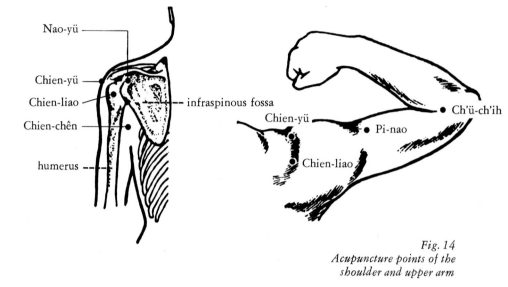

Fig. 14
Acupuncture points of the
shoulder and upper arm

6. Chien-chên, *supra posterior axillary fold (Fig. 14)*

Location. 1.0 inches directly above the posterior axillary fold.
Indications. Painful disorders of the shoulder and upper arm, and paralysis of the upper extremity.
Technique. Perpendicular insertion to a depth of 1.0 to 1.5 inches.
Moxa heating. 5 to 20 minutes.

7. Ch'ü-ch'ih, *lateral antecubital fold (Fig. 14)*

Location. With the forearm flexed and abducted to a horizontal position, the point is located midway between the lateral epicondyle of the humerus and the lateral tip of the antecubital fold.
Indications. Painful disorders of the elbow and upper arm, paralysis of the upper extremity, fever, hypertension, neurodermatitis, pruritus, and other dermatological conditions.
Technique. Perpendicular insertion 0.5 to 1.5 inches deep.
Moxa heating. 5 to 20 minutes.

8. Pi-nao, *mid-humerus (Fig. 14)*

> *Location.* With the forearm flexed and abducted to a horizontal position, the point is located immediately distal to the deltoid muscle, on a line joining the points Chien-yü (UE–2) and Ch'ü-ch'ih (UE–7).
> *Indications.* Painful disorders of the shoulder and upper arm, and paralysis of the upper extremity.
> *Technique.* Perpendicular insertion to a depth of 0.3 to 0.5 inches.
> *Moxa heating.* 5 to 20 minutes.

9. Chi-ch'üan, *axilla (Fig. 15)*

> *Location.* At the center of the axilla.
> *Indications.* Painful disorders of the shoulder and upper arm, and paralysis of the upper extremity.
> *Technique.* Perpendicular insertion to a depth of 0.5 to 1.0 inches.
> *Moxa heating.* 5 to 10 minutes.

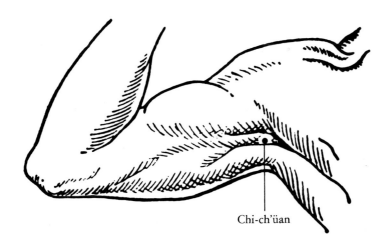

Chi-ch'üan

Fig. 15

10. Chou-liao, *distal humerus (Fig. 16)*

> *Location.* With the forearm flexed and abducted to a horizontal position, the point is located 1.0 inches proximal to Ch'ü-ch'ih (UE–7) on a line drawn from Ch'ü-ch'ih to Chien-yü (UE–2).
> *Indications.* Painful disorders of the elbow.
> *Technique.* Perpendicular insertion along the ventral border of the humerus for a distance of 1.0 to 1.5 inches.
> *Moxa heating.* 5 to 10 minutes.

11. Yang-ch'i, *anatomical snuffbox (Fig. 16)*

> *Location.* With the thumb hyperextended, the point is located in the center of the depression bordered by the tendons of the extensor pollicis longus and brevis, and immediately distal to the styloid process of the radius (anatomical snuffbox).
> *Indications.* Painful disorders of the wrist.
> *Technique.* Perpendicular insertion to a depth of 0.3 to 0.5 inches.
> *Moxa heating.* 10 to 15 minutes.

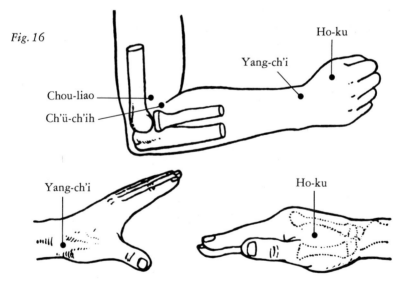

Fig. 16

Ho-ku

Yang-ch'i

Chou-liao

Ch'ü-ch'ih

Yang-ch'i

Ho-ku

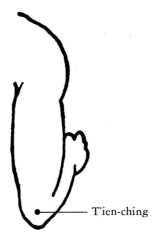

T'ien-ching

Fig. 17

12. Ho-ku, *first dorsal interosseous (Fig. 16)*

Do not use this point in pregnant women.

Location. At the midpoint of a line drawn from the web of the thumb to the confluence of the first and second metacarpals or at the proximal point of the crease formed by approximating the thumb and index finger. It can also be identified by pressing the entire distal phalanx of the thumb against the web of the patient's thumb and locating the point at the tip of the thumb.

Indications. Headache, toothache, pharyngitis, tonsillitis, rhinitis, sinusitis, tinnitus, deafness, eye ailments, induction of labor, menstrual cramps, goiter, painful disorders and paralysis of the upper extremity, neurodermatitis, arthralgia of the mandibular joint, and excessive perspiration.

Technique. With the hand resting on a table, perpendicular insertion to a depth of 0.5 to 1.0 inches.

Moxa heating. 5 to 15 minutes.

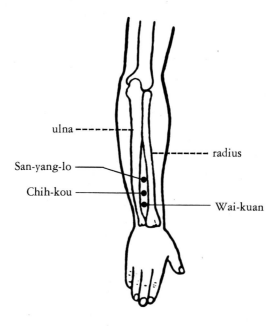

Fig. 18

ulna

radius

San-yang-lo

Chih-kou

Wai-kuan

13. T'ien-ching, *supra olecranon process (Fig. 17)*

Location. 1.0 inches directly proximal to the olecranon process.
Indications. Painful disorders of the elbow.
Technique. Perpendicular insertion 0.5 to 1.0 inches deep.
Moxa heating. 5 to 15 minutes.

14. Chih-kou, *dorsum of mid-forearm (Fig. 18)*

Location. On the dorsum of the forearm 3.0 inches proximal to
the distal tips of the ulna and radius and between these bones.
Indications. Chest pain, shoulder and arm pain, and constipation.
Technique. Perpendicular insertion to depth of 1.0 to 1.5 inches.

15. Wai-kuan, *dorsum of distal forearm (Fig. 18)*

   Location. On the dorsum of the forearm, 2.0 inches proximal to the distal tips of the ulna and radius and between these bones.
   Indications. Paralysis of the upper extremity, chest pain, headaches, deafness, tinnitus, torticollis, and influenza.
   Technique. Perpendicular insertion 0.8 to 1.5 inches deep.
   Moxa heating. 5 to 15 minutes.

16. Yang-ch'ih, *dorsum of wrist (Fig. 19)*

   Location. On the dorsum of the wrist, in line with the confluence of the third and fourth metacarpals.
   Indications. Painful disorders of the wrist.
   Technique. Perpendicular insertion 0.2 to 0.3 inches deep.
   Moxa heating. 5 to 10 minutes.

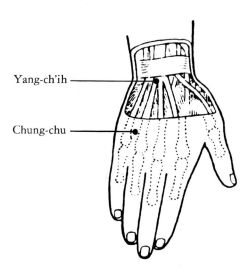

Yang-ch'ih

Chung-chu

Fig. 19

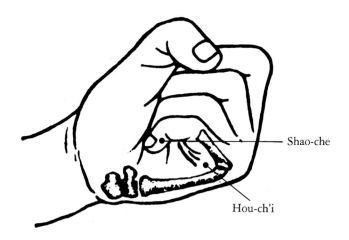

Shao-che

Hou-ch'i

Fig. 20

17. Chung-chu, *inter fourth and fifth metacarpals (Fig. 19)*

Location. On the dorsum of the hand, between the fourth and fifth metacarpals and 0.5 inches proximal to the corresponding metacarpo-phalangeal joints.
Indications. Tinnitus, deafness, mutism, headaches, pharyngitis, and rigidity of the fingers.
Technique. Perpendicular insertion to a depth of 0.5 to 0.8 inches.
Moxa heating. 5 to 10 minutes.

18. Hou-ch'i, *distal fifth metacarpal (Fig. 20)*

Location. With the hand making a fist, the point is located at the medial tip of the major palmar crease, immediately ventral to the distal portion of the fifth metacarpal.
Indications. Occipital headaches, backaches, tinnitus, torticollis, and finger spasm and numbness.
Technique. Perpendicular insertion 0.5 to 1.0 inches deep.
Moxa heating. 5 to 15 minutes.

19. Shao-che, *fifth fingernail (Fig. 20)*

   Location. At the intersection of the base and the ulnar margin of the fingernail of the fifth finger.
   Indications. Insufficiency of lactation, mastitis, and headaches.
   Technique. Diagonal insertion toward the interphalangeal joint to a depth of 0.1 inches.
   Moxa heating. 5 to 15 minutes.

20. Ch'ih-che, *antecubital fossa (Fig. 21)*

   Location. In the antecubital fossa immediately lateral to the tendon of the biceps. The point is best identified with the forearm in slight flexion.
   Indications. Painful disorders of the elbow, cough, and pharyngitis.
   Technique. Perpendicular insertion 0.5 to 1.0 inches deep.
   Moxa heating. 5 to 10 minutes.

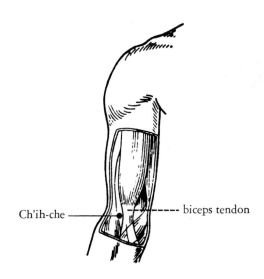

Ch'ih-che ———— •---- biceps tendon

Fig. 21

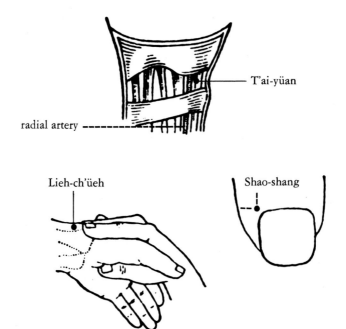

radial artery ----------

T'ai-yüan

Lieh-ch'üeh

Shao-shang

Fig. 22

21. Lieh-ch'üeh, *proximal to styloid process of radius (Fig. 22)*

Location. Immediately proximal to the styloid process of the radius or 2 fingers' width proximal to the anatomical snuffbox (see Yang-ch'i, UE–11) between the tendons of the abductor pollicis longus and the brachioradialis. It can also be located at the tip of the index finger of the opposite hand when the webs between the thumb and index finger of both hands are interlocked.

Indications. Painful disorders of the wrist, cough, and headache of the vertex of the head.

Technique. Diagonal insertion in the direction of the elbow, 0.5 to 1.0 inches deep.

22. T'ai-yüan, *lateral ventral wrist (Fig. 22)*

   Location. Between the tendon of the abductor pollicis longus and
   the radial artery, at the level of the most distal crease on the ventral
   surface of the wrist.
   Indications. Painful disorders of the wrist, cough, dypsnea, and
   pharyngitis.
   Technique. Perpendicular insertion 0.2 to 0.3 inches deep.

23. Shao-shang, *thumbnail (Fig. 22)*

   Location. At the intersection of the radial margin and the base of
   the thumbnail.
   Indications. Cough, pharyngitis, tonsillitis, and syncope.
   Technique. Diagonal insertion towards the base of the thumb 0.1
   to 0.2 inches deep. This point is also for blood-letting in cases of
   syncope.
   Moxa heating. 1 to 3 minutes.

24. Hsi-mên, *ventral forearm #1 (Fig. 23)*

   Location. 5.0 inches proximal to the most distal crease of the wrist,
   on the ventral surface of the forearm and between the tendons of
   the flexor carpi radialis and palmaris longus.
   Indications. Palpitations and angina pectoris.
   Technique. Perpendicular insertion 0.5 to 1.5 inches deep.
   Moxa heating. 5 to 15 minutes.

25. Chien-shih, *ventral forearm #2 (Fig. 23)*

   Location. 3.0 inches proximal to the most distal crease of the wrist,
   on the ventral surface of the forearm and between the tendons of
   the flexor carpi radialis and palmaris longus.
   Indications. Palpitations, angina pectoris, epilepsy, mental disorders, and malaria.

Technique. Perpendicular insertion to a depth of 0.5 to 1.5 inches.
Moxa heating. 5 to 15 minutes.

26. Nei-kuan, *ventral forearm #3 (Fig. 23)*

Location. 2.0 inches proximal to the most distal crease of the wrist
on the ventral surface of the forearm and between the tendons of
the flexor carpi radialis and palmaris longus.
Indications. Abdominal pain, epigastric pain, emesis, palpitations,
angina pectoris, chest pain, numbness of the forearm and fingers,
and malaria.
Technique. Perpendicular insertion 0.5 to 1.0 inches deep.
Moxa heating. 5 to 15 minutes.

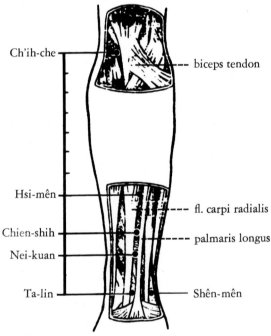

Ch'ih-che — biceps tendon

Hsi-mên — fl. carpi radialis

Chien-shih — palmaris longus

Nei-kuan —

Ta-lin — Shên-mên

Fig. 23
Acupuncture points of the
forearm, ventral surface

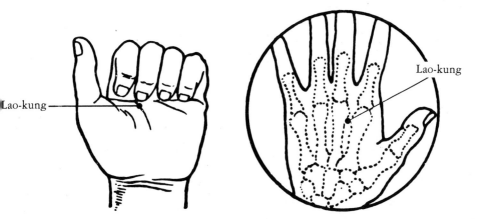

Fig. 24

27. Ta-lin, *midpoint of ventral wrist (Fig. 23)*

    Location. Immediately proximal to the most distal crease on the ventral surface of the wrist and between the tendons of the flexor carpi radialis and palmaris longus.
    Indications. Painful disorders of the wrist and palpitations.
    Technique. Perpendicular insertion 0.3 to 0.5 inches deep.
    Moxa heating. 5 to 15 minutes.

28. Lao-kung, *distal third metacarpal (Fig. 24)*
    Location. On the palm, 1.0 inches from the third metacarpophalangeal joint, between the second and third metacarpals. It can also be located at the point where the tip of the completely flexed middle finger touches the most distal major palmar crease.
    Indications. Dermatitis of the hand and stomatitis.
    Technique. Perpendicular insertion 0.3 to 0.5 inches deep.
    Moxa heating. 5 to 10 minutes.

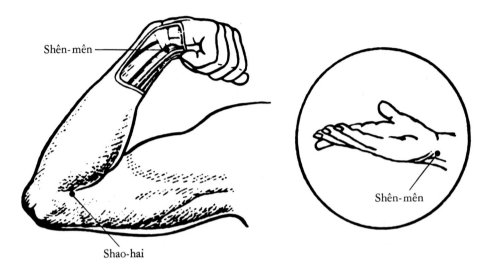

Shên-mên

Shao-hai

Shên-mên

Fig. 25

29. Shao-hai, *medial antecubital fold (Fig. 25)*

   Location. At the medial tip of the antecubital fold when the forearm is completely flexed.
   Indications. Painful disorders of the elbow.
   Technique. Perpendicular insertion 0.5 to 1.0 inches deep.
   Moxa heating. 5 to 10 minutes.

30. Shên-mên, *medial aspect of ventral wrist (Fig. 25)*

   Location. At the most distal crease on the ventral surface of the wrist, immediately proximal to the pisiform bone and medial to the tendon of the flexor carpi ulnaris.
   Indications. Insomnia, palpitations, and neurasthenia.
   Technique. Perpendicular insertion 0.3 to 0.5 inches deep.
   Moxa heating. 5 to 15 minutes.

31. Pa-hsieh, *inter metacarpo-phalangeal joints (Fig. 26)*

    Location. With the hand making a fist, the points are located 0.5 inches proximal to the webs of the fingers.

    Indications. Painful disorders and numbness of the fingers and finger joints, headache, toothache, pharyngitis, and painful disorders of the neck.

    Technique. With the hand loosely clenched, perpendicular insertion, parallel to the metacarpals, approximately 0.5 inches deep.

32. Shang-pa-hsieh, *inter distal metacarpals (Fig. 26)*

    Location. Between the distal portions of the metacarpals and immediately proximal to the metacarpo-phalangeal joints. The point between the first and second metacarpals corresponds to the point Ho-ku (UE–12) while the point between the fourth and fifth metacarpals is similar to the point Chung-chu (UE–17).

    Indications. Painful disorders and numbness of the fingers and finger joints, headache, toothache, pharyngitis, and painful disorders of the neck.

    Technique. Perpendicular insertion to a depth of 0.3 to 0.5 inches.

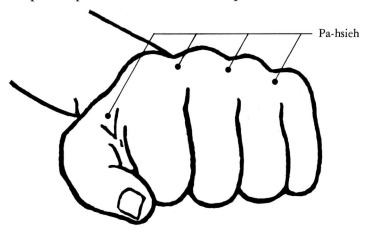
Pa-hsieh

Fig. 26

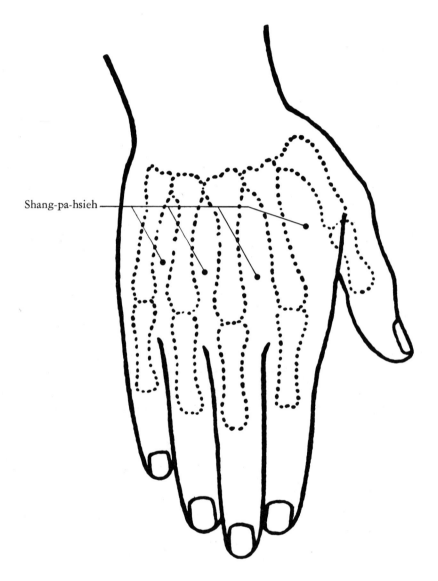

Shang-pa-hsieh

Fig. 26

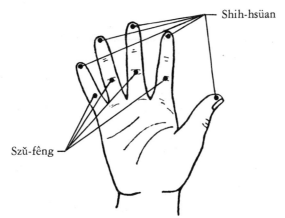

Shih-hsüan

Szŭ-fêng

Fig. 27

33. Szŭ-fêng, *proximal interphalangeal joints (Fig. 27)*

Location. At the ventral surface of the second to the fifth proximal interphalangeal joints.
Indications. Pediatric digestive disorders and pertussis.
Technique. Perpendicular insertion 0.1 inches deep. This should produce the escape of a yellowish, transparent fluid.

34. Shih-hsüan, *fingertips (Fig. 27)*

Location. At the tip of each finger and 0.1 inches below the finger-nail.
Indications. Syncope and shock.
Technique. Puncture each point till blood is produced (blood-letting).

35. San-yang-lo *(Fig. 18)*

Location. On the dorsum of the forearm, 4.0 inches proximal to the distal end of the ulna and radius and between these bones.
Indications. Deafness, laryngitis, and painful disorders of the arm.
Technique. Perpendicular insertion 0.5 to 1.0 inches deep.
Moxa heating. 5 to 20 minutes.

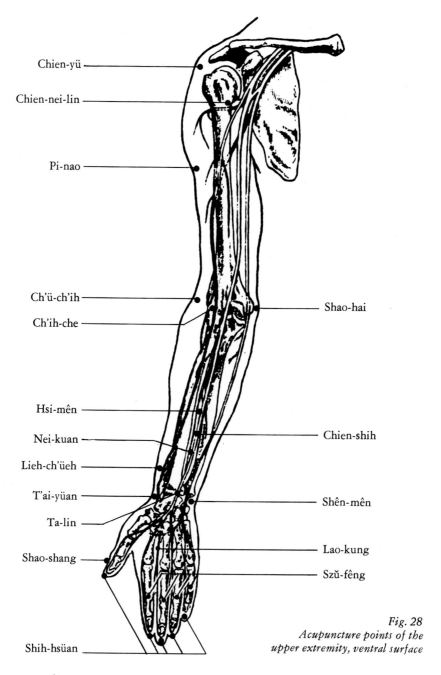

Chien-yü

Chien-nei-lin

Pi-nao

Ch'ü-ch'ih

Ch'ih-che

Shao-hai

Hsi-mên

Nei-kuan

Chien-shih

Lieh-ch'üeh

T'ai-yüan

Shên-mên

Ta-lin

Shao-shang

Lao-kung

Szŭ-fêng

Shih-hsüan

Fig. 28
Acupuncture points of the
upper extremity, ventral surface

62

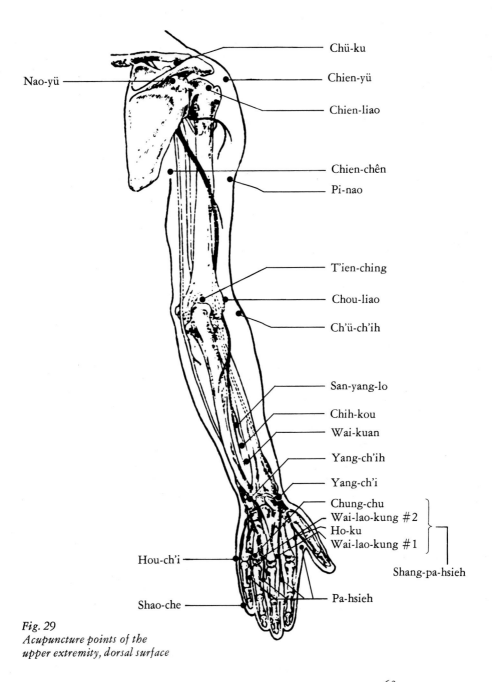

Chü-ku

Chien-yü

Chien-liao

Nao-yü

Chien-chên

Pi-nao

T'ien-ching

Chou-liao

Ch'ü-ch'ih

San-yang-lo

Chih-kou

Wai-kuan

Yang-ch'ih

Yang-ch'i

Chung-chu
Wai-lao-kung #2
Ho-ku
Wai-lao-kung #1

Hou-ch'i

Shao-che

Pa-hsieh

Shang-pa-hsieh

Fig. 29
Acupuncture points of the
upper extremity, dorsal surface

Table 2

SUMMARY OF ACUPUNCTURE POINTS OF THE UPPER EXTREMITY

LOCATION	NAME	COMMON INDICATIONS	SPECIFIC INDICATIONS
Shoulder	Chü-ku Chien-yü Chien-nei-lin Chien-chên Nao-yü Chi-ch'üan Pi-nao	Painful disorders of the shoulder, paralysis of the upper extremity	
Arm and hand, dorsal surface	Chou-liao Ch'ü-ch'ih Yang-ch'i Ho-ku	Diseases of the head and throat — Diseases of the eye, ear, nose, and mouth	Chou-liao: Painful disorders of the elbow Ch'ü-ch'ih: Painful disorders of the elbow, hypertension, pruritus Yang-ch'i: Painful disorders of the wrist Ho-ku: Deafness, tinnitus, induction of labor, excessive perspiration, painful disorders of the mandibular joint
	T'ien-ching Chih-kou Wai-kuan Yang-ch'ih Chung-chu San-yang-lo	Diseases of the eye, malar, maxilla, mandible and chest	T'ien-ching: Painful disorders of the elbow Chih-kou: Constipation Wai-kuan: Torticollis, influenza Yang-ch'ih: Painful disorders of the wrist

	Hou-ch'i Shao-che		Hou-ch'i: Backache, finger spasm and numbness Shao-che: Diseases of the breast
	Ch'ih-che Lieh-ch'üeh T'ai-yüan Shao-shang	Diseases of the throat and lung	Ch'ih-che: Painful disorders of the elbow Lieh-ch'üeh: Headache, painful disorders of the wrist T'ai-yüan: Painful disorders of the wrist Shao-shang: Syncope
Arm and hand, ventral surface	Hsi-mên Chien-shih Nei-kuan Ta-lin Lao-kung	Diseases of the chest Diseases of the heart	Chien-shih: Epilepsy, malaria Nei-kuan: Painful disorders of the stomach and intestine, malaria Ta-lin: Painful disorders of the wrist Lao-kung: Stomatitis, dermatitis of the hand
	Shao-hai Shên-mên		Shao-hai: Painful disorders of the elbow Shên-mên: Insomnia
Hand, dorsum	Pa-hsieh Shang-pa-hsieh	Painful disorders and numbness of the fingers	
Hand, ventral surface	Szŭ-fêng Shih-hsüan		Szŭ-fêng: Pediatric digestive disorders, pertussis Shih-hsüan: Syncope

POINTS OF THE LOWER EXTREMITY

1. Huan-t'iao, *posterior hip (Fig. 30)*

Location. With the patient lying in a lateral position and with the knees partially flexed, the point is located at one-third the distance of a line drawn from the greater trochanter of the femur to the base of the coccyx.

Indications. Sciatica, paralysis of the lower extremity, and painful disorders of the hip.

Technique. Perpendicular insertion 2.0 to 3.0 inches deep.

Moxa heating. 10 to 30 minutes.

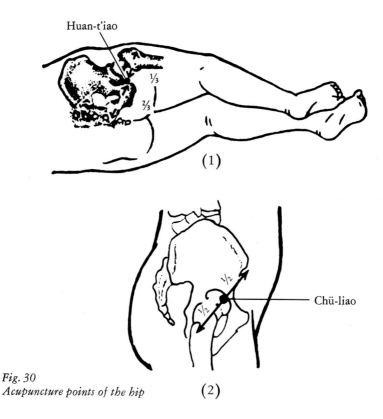

Fig. 30
Acupuncture points of the hip

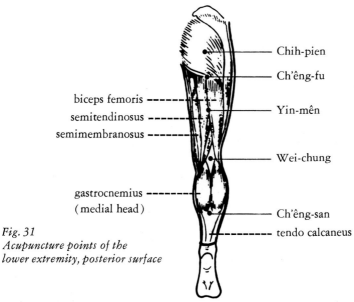

Chih-pien

Ch'êng-fu

biceps femoris ------
semitendinosus ------
semimembranosus ------

Yin-mên

Wei-chung

gastrocnemius --------
(medial head)

Ch'êng-san
tendo calcaneus

Fig. 31
Acupuncture points of the
lower extremity, posterior surface

2. Chü-liao, *lateral hip (Fig. 30)*

Location. With the patient lying in a lateral position and with the knees partially flexed, it is at the midpoint of a line drawn from the anterior superior iliac spine to the greater trochanter of the femur.
Indications. Painful disorders of the hip and lower extremity.
Technique. Perpendicular insertion 2.0 to 3.0 inches deep.
Moxa heating. 5 to 20 minutes.

3. Ch'êng-fu, *gluteal fold (Fig. 31)*

Location. At the midline on the posterior surface of the thigh and at the level of the gluteal fold.
Indications. Sciatica, paralysis of the lower extremity, hemorrhoids, renal failure, and low back pain.
Technique. Perpendicular insertion 1.5 to 2.5 inches deep.
Moxa heating. 5 to 20 minutes.

4. Yin-lien, *base of femoral triangle (Fig. 32)*

Location. 1.0 inches distal to the inguinal ligament and immediately lateral to the femoral artery.
Indications. Low back pain, and paralysis and pain of the lower extremity.
Technique. Perpendicular insertion 1.0 to 1.5 inches deep.
Moxa heating. 5 to 10 minutes.

5. Fu-t'u, *anterior mid-thigh (Fig. 32)*

Location. On the anterior surface of the thigh, 6.0 inches directly proximal to the lateral edge of the base of the patella. The distance of the point from the base of the patella is equivalent to the length of the patient's hand.
Indications. Paralysis of the lower extremity and painful disorders of the knee.
Technique. Perpendicular insertion along the lateral edge of the femur to a depth of 2.0 to 3.0 inches.
Moxa heating. 5 to 20 minutes.

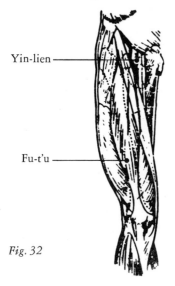

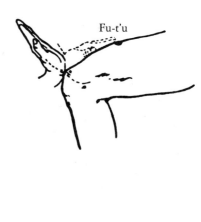

Fu-t'u

Yin-lien

Fu-t'u

Fig. 32

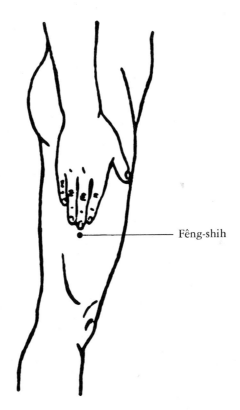

Fêng-shih

Fig. 33

6. Fêng-shih, *lateral mid-thigh (Fig. 33)*

Location. At the midline on the lateral aspect of the thigh, 7.0 inches directly proximal to a line at the level of the base of the patella. With the patient standing erect and his arm hanging at his side, the point can also be located immediately distal to the tip of the middle finger on the lateral surface of the thigh.

Indications. Paralysis and pain of the lower extremity, low back pain, and neurodermatitis of the lateral aspect of the thigh.

Technique. Perpendicular insertion 1.5 to 2.5 inches deep.

Moxa heating. 5 to 20 minutes.

7. Yin-mên, *posterior mid-thigh (Fig. 31)*

Location. At the midline on the posterior aspect of the thigh, 6.0 inches directly distal to the point Ch'êng-fu (LE–3) or to the gluteal fold.
Indications. Sciatica, lumbago, and paralysis of the lower extremity.
Technique. Perpendicular insertion 1.5 to 3.0 inches deep.
Moxa heating. 5 to 20 minutes.

8. Nei-wai-ch'i-yen, *para ligament patellae (Fig. 34)*

Location. In the joint space on each side of the ligament patellae.
Indications. Painful disorders of the knee.
Technique. Perpendicular insertion 1.5 to 2.0 inches deep.
Moxa heating. 5 to 15 minutes.

9. Liang-ch'iu, *supra lateral patella (Fig. 34)*

Location. 2.0 inches directly proximal to the lateral edge of the base of the patella.
Indications. Painful disorders of the knee, numbness of the lower extremity, and gastralgia.
Technique. Perpendicular insertion to a depth of 1.0 to 1.5 inches.
Moxa heating. 5 to 15 minutes.

10. Tsu-san-li, *pretibial #1 (Fig. 34)*

Location. 3.0 inches directly distal to the point where the lateral and apical (distal) margins of the patella meet. It can also be located at a point 1.0 inches distal and lateral to the tibial tubercle (tuberosity).
Indications. Abdominal pain, gastralgia, diarrhea, gastro-intestinal complaints, hypertension, malaise, fatigue, anemia, paralysis of the lower extremity, and painful disorders of the knee.
Technique. Perpendicular insertion 1.0 to 2.0 inches deep.
Moxa heating. 10 to 30 minutes.

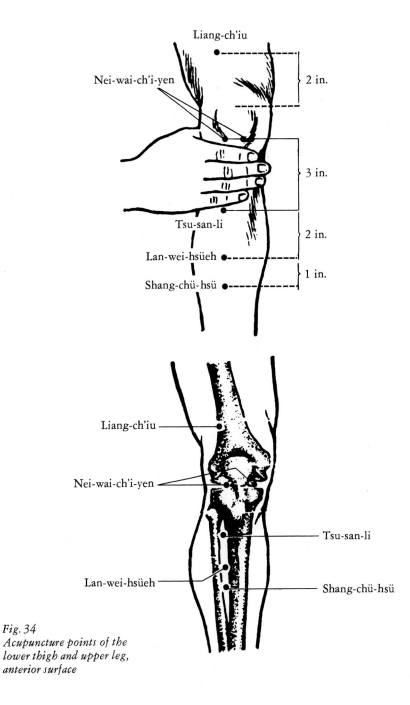

Liang-ch'iu

Nei-wai-ch'i-yen

2 in.

3 in.

Tsu-san-li

2 in.

Lan-wei-hsüeh

1 in.

Shang-chü-hsü

Liang-ch'iu

Nei-wai-ch'i-yen

Tsu-san-li

Lan-wei-hsüeh

Shang-chü-hsü

Fig. 34
Acupuncture points of the
lower thigh and upper leg,
anterior surface

11. Lan-wei-hsüeh, *pretibial #2 or appendix point (Fig. 34)*

Location. 2.0 inches directly distal to the point Tsu-san-li (LE–10). When appendicitis is present, point tenderness will be elicited when digital pressure is applied on the point.
Indications. Appendicitis.
Technique. Perpendicular insertion 1.5 to 2.0 inches deep.

12. Shang-chü-hsü, *pretibial #3 (Fig. 34)*

Location. 6.0 inches directly distal to the point where the lateral and apical (distal) margins of the patella intersect and 1.0 inches lateral to the tibia. It is also 1.0 inches distal to the point Lan-wei-hsüeh (LE–11).
Indications. Abdominal pain, diarrhea, and appendicitis.
Technique. Perpendicular insertion 1.0 to 2.0 inches deep.
Moxa heating. 5 to 20 minutes.

13. Chiai-ch'i, *dorsum of ankle (Fig. 35)*

Location. Directly in line with the second toe, in the groove between the tendons of the tibialis anterior and the extensor hallucis longus at the level of the center of the medial malleolus.
Indications. Painful disorders of the ankle, and paralysis of the lower extremity.
Technique. Perpendicular insertion, in the direction of the calcaneum, 0.5 to 1.0 inches deep.
Moxa heating. 5 to 10 minutes.

14. Nei-t'ing, *inter second and third metatarsals (Fig. 35)*

Location. On the dorsum of the foot between the second and third metatarsals and one index finger's width proximal to the corresponding metatarso-phalangeal joints.

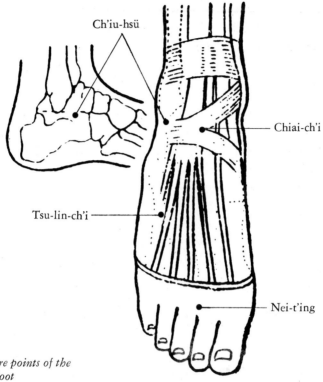

Ch'iu-hsü

Chiai-ch'i

Tsu-lin-ch'i

Nei-t'ing

Fig. 35
Acupuncture points of the
ankle and foot

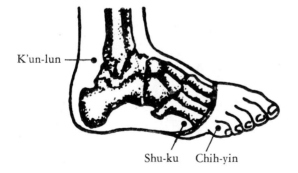

K'un-lun

Shu-ku   Chih-yin

Indications. Toothache, tonsillitis, tic douloureux, and headache.
Technique. Diagonal insertion towards the calcaneum to a depth of 0.2 to 0.5 inches.
Moxa heating. 5 to 10 minutes.

15. Yang-lin-ch'üan, *anterior to neck of fibula (Fig. 36)*

Location. Immediately anterior to the neck of the fibula.
Indications. Rib pain, diseases of the gallbladder and bile ducts, paralysis of the lower extremity, and painful disorders of the knee.
Technique. Perpendicular insertion to a depth of 0.5 to 2.0 inches.
Moxa heating. 5 to 15 minutes.

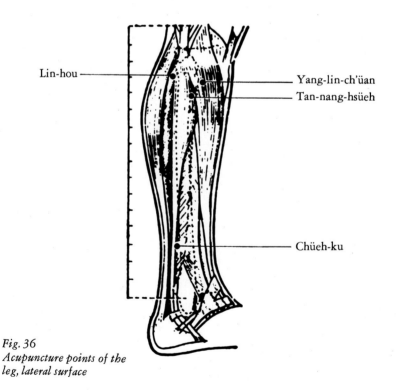

Lin-hou

Yang-lin-ch'üan
Tan-nang-hsüeh

Chüeh-ku

Fig. 36
Acupuncture points of the leg, lateral surface

74

16. Tan-nang-hsüeh, *proximal fibula or gallbladder point (Fig. 36)*

Location. Between 1.0 to 2.0 inches directly distal to the point for Yang-lin-ch'üan (LE–15). In a patient afflicted with pain from diseases of the gallbladder and bile ducts, point tenderness will be elicited upon applying digital pressure on the point.
Indications. Diseases of the gallbladder and bile ducts.
Technique. Perpendicular insertion to a depth of 1.0 to 2.0 inches.

17. Chüeh-ku, *distal fibula (Fig. 36)*

Location. 3.0 inches proximal to the lateral malleolus and between the fibula and the tendon of the peroneus longus.
Indications. Paralysis of the lower extremity, torticollis, and painful disorders of the ankle.
Technique. Perpendicular insertion 1.0 to 2.0 inches deep.
Moxa heating. 5 to 10 minutes.

18. Ch'iu-hsü, *lateral malleolus (Fig. 35)*

Location. At the point where the anterior and distal margins of the lateral malleolus intersect.
Indications. Painful disorders of the ankle, and rib pain.
Technique. Perpendicular insertion 1.0 to 1.5 inches deep.
Moxa heating. 5 to 10 minutes.

19. Tsu-lin-ch'i, *inter fourth and fifth metatarsals (Fig. 35)*

Location. On the dorsum of the foot between the fourth and fifth metatarsals and immediately lateral to the tendon of the extensor digitorum longus.
Indications. Suppression of lactation, mastitis, rib pain, headache, dizziness, and foot pain.
Technique. Perpendicular insertion 0.3 to 0.5 inches deep.
Moxa heating. 5 to 10 minutes.

20. Wei-chung, *popliteal fossa (Fig. 31)*

   Location. At the center of the popliteal fossa.
   Indications. Sciatica, lumbago, paralysis of the lower extremity,
   Technique. Perpendicular insertion 0.5 to 1.0 inches deep. This is
   also a point for blood-letting.
   Moxa heating. 3 to 5 minutes.

21. Ch'êng-san, *gastrocnemius (Fig. 31)*

   Location. At the distal margin of the gastrocnemius muscle and
   between its medial and lateral heads. Hyperextension of the lower
   extremity will accentuate the outline of the muscle.
   Indications. Sciatica, rectal prolapse, spasm of the gastrocnemius
   muscle, paralysis of the lower extremity, and pain of the sole of
   the foot.
   Technique. Perpendicular insertion 1.0 to 2.5 inches deep.
   Moxa heating. 5 to 15 minutes.

22. K'un-lun, *posterior to lateral malleolus (Fig. 35)*

   Location. Midpoint between the posterior margin of the lateral
   malleolus and the Achilles tendon.
   Indications. Paralysis of the lower extremity, sciatica, and painful
   disorders of the ankle.
   Technique. Perpendicular insertion 0.5 inches deep.
   Moxa heating. 5 to 15 minutes.

23. Shu-ku, *fifth metatarsal (Fig. 35)*

   Location. Immediately beneath the fifth metatarsal and proximal
   to the fifth metatarso-phalangeal joint.
   Indications. Headache, dizziness, and low back pain.
   Technique. Perpendicular insertion 0.3 to 0.5 inches deep.
   Moxa heating. 5 to 10 minutes.

24. Chih-yin, *base of fifth toenail (Fig. 35)*

> *Location.* At the point where the lateral and proximal margins of the fifth toenail intersect.
> *Indications.* Malposition of fetus and headache.
> *Technique.* Diagonal insertion towards the base of the toe to a depth of 0.1 to 0.2 inches.
> *Moxa heating.* 10 to 30 minutes.

25. Hsüeh-hai, *medial supra patella (Fig. 37)*

> *Location.* At the center of the distal portion of the vastus medialis muscle, at a level 2.0 inches proximal to the patella. With the knee in 90° flexion, the practitioner, by cupping his hand over the patient's patella, can also locate the point immediately distal to the tip of his thumb.
> *Indications.* Neurodermatitis, hives, pruritus, and menstrual irregularities.
> *Technique.* Perpendicular insertion 1.0 to 2.0 inches deep.
> *Moxa heating.* 5 to 15 minutes.

26. Yin-lin-ch'üan, *posterior proximal tibia (Fig. 37)*

> *Location.* At the posterior edge of the tibia and immediately distal to its medial condyle. It is at the level of and opposite the point Yang-lin-ch'üan (LE–15).
> *Indications.* Abdominal distention, diarrhea, menstrual irregularity, urinary retention, edema, and painful disorders of the knee.
> *Technique.* Perpendicular insertion 1.0 to 3.0 inches deep.
> *Moxa heating.* 5 to 15 minutes.

27. San-yin-chiao, *posterior to distal tibia (Fig. 38)*

> Do not use this point in pregnant women.

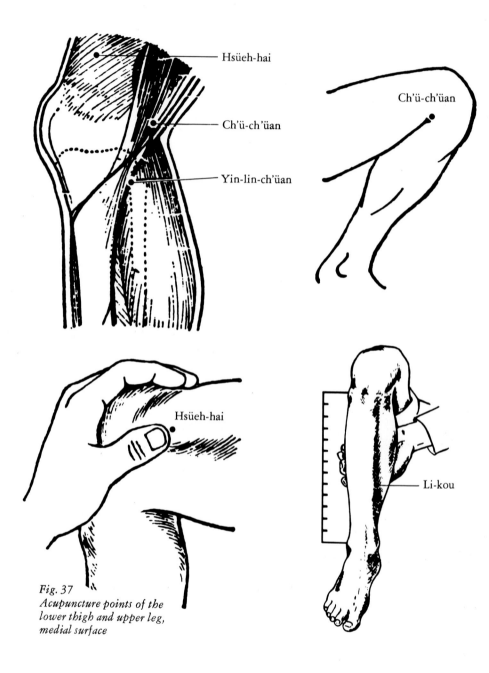

Hsüeh-hai

Ch'ü-ch'üan

Yin-lin-ch'üan

Ch'ü-ch'üan

Hsüeh-hai

Li-kou

Fig. 37
*Acupuncture points of the
lower thigh and upper leg,
medial surface*

Location. 3.0 inches proximal to the medial malleolus and immediately posterior to the tibia.
Indications. Urological and gynecological disorders, neurasthenia, lower abdominal pain, diarrhea, insomnia, neurodermatitis, pruritus, and hives.
Technique. Perpendicular insertion 0.5 to 1.5 inches deep.
Moxa heating. 10 to 20 minutes.

28. Shang-ch'iu, *medial malleolus (Fig. 38)*

Location. At the point where the anterior and distal margins of the medial malleolus intersect.
Indications. Painful disorders of the ankle and indigestion.
Technique. Perpendicular insertion 0.3 to 0.5 inches deep.
Moxa heating. 5 to 20 minutes.

29. Kung-sun, *first metatarsal (Fig. 38)*

Location. Immediately beneath the first metatarsal and 1.0 inches proximal to the first metatarso-phalangeal joint.
Indications. Gastralgia, abdominal pain, and diarrhea.
Technique. Perpendicular insertion 0.7 to 1.0 inches deep.
Moxa heating. 5 to 15 minutes.

30. Yin-pê, *first toenail (Fig. 38)*

Location. At the intersection of the medial margin and the base of the first toenail.
Indications. Menorrhagia, uterine bleeding, and abdominal pain.
Technique. Diagonal insertion towards the base of the toe 0.1 to 0.2 inches deep.
Moxa heating. 5 to 20 minutes.

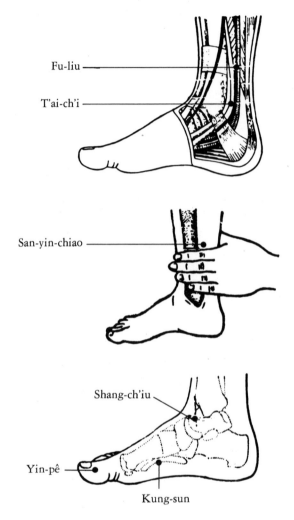

Fu-liu

T'ai-ch'i

San-yin-chiao

Shang-ch'iu

Yin-pê

Kung-sun

Fig. 38
Acupuncture points of the
lower leg and foot,
medial surface

31. Ch'ü-ch'üan, *medial popliteal fold (Fig. 37)*

Location. At the medial tip of the popliteal fold when the knee is flexed.
Indications. Nocturnal emission, dysuria, impotence, and painful disorders of the knee.
Technique. Perpendicular insertion 1.0 to 1.5 inches deep.
Moxa heating. 5 to 15 minutes.

32. Li-kou, *posterior to mid-tibia (Fig. 37)*

Location. 5.0 inches proximal to the medial malleolus and immediately posterior to the tibia.
Indications. Pelvic inflammatory diseases, renal failure, nocturnal emission, and impotence.
Technique. Perpendicular insertion 0.5 to 1.0 inches deep.
Moxa heating. 3 to 5 minutes.

33. T'ai-ch'ung, *inter first and second metatarsals (Fig. 39)*

Location. Between the first and second metatarsals and 2.0 inches proximal to the corresponding metatarso-phalangeal joints.
Indications. Headache, dizziness, hypertension, metrorrhagia, and mastitis.
Technique. Diagonal insertion towards the calcaneum 0.5 to 1.0 inches deep.
Moxa heating. 5 to 15 minutes.

34. T'ai-ch'i, *posterior to medial malleolus (Fig. 38)*

Location. On the medial surface of the ankle, at the midpoint of a line drawn from the posterior border of the medial malleolus to the Achilles tendon.
Indications. Low backache, hematuria, disorders of the reproduc-

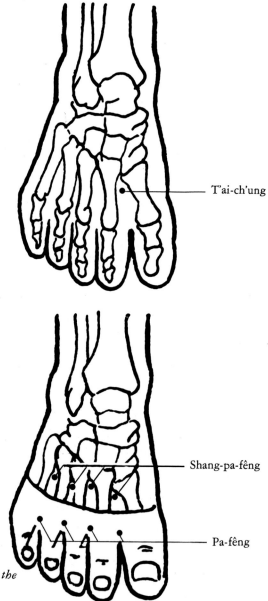

T'ai-ch'ung

Shang-pa-fêng

Pa-fêng

Fig. 39
Acupuncture points of the
foot, dorsal surface

tive system, pain of the sole of the foot, paralysis of the lower extremity, and nervous breakdown.
Technique. Perpendicular insertion 0.3 to 0.5 inches deep.
Moxa heating. 5 to 15 minutes.

35. Fu-liu, *posterior to distal tibia (Fig. 38)*

Location. 2.0 inches directly proximal to the point T'ai-ch'i (LE–34).
Indications. Edema, excessive perspiration, and paralysis of the lower extremity.
Technique. Perpendicular insertion to a depth of 1.0 to 1.5 inches.
Moxa heating. 5 to 20 minutes.

36. Yung-ch'üan, *sole of foot (Fig. 40)*

Location. At the midline of the sole of the foot at a point one-third the distance of a line drawn from the third metatarso-phalangeal joint to the heel.
Indications. Headache, sun-stroke, and shock.
Technique. Perpendicular insertion 0.5 to 1.0 inches deep.
Moxa heating. 5 to 10 minutes.

37. Pa-fêng, *inter metatarso-phalangeal joints (Fig. 39)*

Location. 0.5 inches proximal to the web of the toes.
Indications. Pain, numbness, and inflammatory conditions of the dorsum of the foot and the toes.
Technique. Perpendicular insertion 0.5 inches deep.
Moxa heating. 5 to 10 minutes.

38. Shang-pa-fêng, *inter proximal metatarsals (Fig. 39)*

Location. Between the metatarsals and immediately distal to their bases.

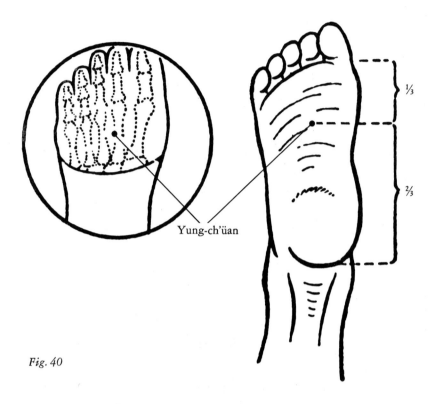

Yung-ch'üan

Fig. 40

Indications. Pain, numbness, and inflammatory conditions of the dorsum of the foot and the toes.
Technique. Perpendicular insertion 0.5 to 1.0 inches deep.
Moxa heating. 5 to 15 minutes.

39. Lin-hou, *posterior to neck of fibula (Fig. 36)*

Location. Immediately posterior to the neck of the fibula.
Indications. Sciatica and paralysis of the lower extremity.
Technique. Perpendicular insertion to a depth of 0.3 to 0.5 inches.
Moxa heating. 5 to 15 minutes.

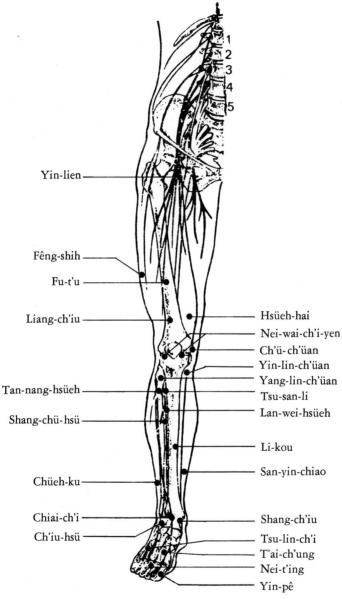

Yin-lien

Fêng-shih

Fu-t'u

Liang-ch'iu

Tan-nang-hsüeh

Shang-chü-hsü

Chüeh-ku

Chiai-ch'i

Ch'iu-hsü

Hsüeh-hai

Nei-wai-ch'i-yen

Ch'ü-ch'üan

Yin-lin-ch'üan

Yang-lin-ch'üan

Tsu-san-li

Lan-wei-hsüeh

Li-kou

San-yin-chiao

Shang-ch'iu

Tsu-lin-ch'i

T'ai-ch'ung

Nei-t'ing

Yin-pê

Fig. 41
Acupuncture points of the
lower extremity, anterior surface

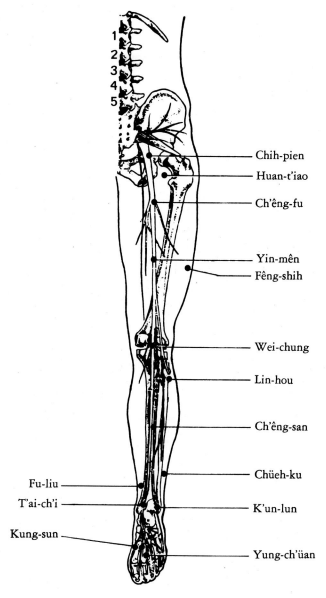

1
2
3
4
5

Chih-pien
Huan-t'iao
Ch'êng-fu

Yin-mên
Fêng-shih

Wei-chung

Lin-hou

Ch'êng-san

Chüeh-ku

K'un-lun

Yung-ch'üan

Fu-liu
T'ai-ch'i
Kung-sun

Fig. 42
Acupuncture points of the
lower extremity, posterior surface

87

Table 3

SUMMARY OF ACUPUNCTURE POINTS OF LOWER EXTREMITY

LOCATION	NAME	COMMON INDICATIONS		SPECIFIC INDICATIONS
Hip	Huan-t'iao Chü-liao	Painful disorders of the hip	Paralysis of the lower extremity, hip-joint pain	Huan-t'iao: Sciatica, paralysis of the lower extremities
	Ch'êng-fu Yin-mên	Sciatica		Ch'êng-fu: Renal failure, acute Yin-mên: Lumbago
	Fêng-shih			Fêng-shih: Neurodermatitis of the thigh, lateral surface
Thigh	Yin-lien Fu-t'u	Disorders of the anterior surface of the thigh		Yin-lien: Painful disorders of the back and leg Fu-t'u: Painful disorders of the knee
Knee	Nei-wai-ch'i-yen		Diseases of the head and local area, paralysis of lower extremity	Painful disorders of the knee
Leg and Foot	Liang-ch'iu Tsu-san-li Lan-wei-hsüeh Shang-chü-hsü Chiai-ch'i Nei-t'ing	Diseases of the face, stomach, and intestines		Liang-ch'iu: Painful disorders of the knee Tsu-san-li: Hypertension, anemia, chronic fatigue Lan-wei-hsüeh: Appendicitis Shang-chü-hsü: Inflammation of the intestine Chiai-ch'i: Painful disorders of the ankle Nei-t'ing: Tonsillitis

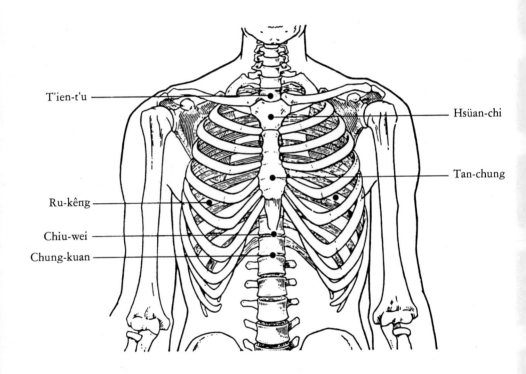

T'ien-t'u

Hsüan-chi

Tan-chung

Ru-kêng

Chiu-wei

Chung-kuan

Fig. 43
Acupuncture points of the chest

POINTS OF THE CHEST AND ABDOMEN

1. T'ien-t'u, *supra sternal notch (Figs. 43 and 44)*

Location. With the neck hyperextended, the point is located 0.5 inches superior to the sternal notch of the sternum.
Indications. Asthma, upper respiratory infections, pharyngitis, and diaphragmodynia.
Technique. Horizontal insertion, caudad behind the sternum, to a depth of 0.5 to 0.7 inches.
Moxa heating. 5 to 15 minutes.

2. Hsüan-chi, *manubrium sterni (Figs. 43 and 44)*

Location. 1.0 inches directly inferior to the point T'ien-t'u (CA–1).
Indications. Asthma.
Technique. Horizontal insertion, caudad, 0.5 to 1.0 inches deep.
Moxa heating. 5 to 15 minutes.

3. Tan-chung, *xiphi-sternal junction (Figs. 43 and 44)*

Location. At the xiphi-sternal junction, midpoint between the nipples.
Indications. Asthma, upper respiratory infections, and insufficiency of lactation.
Technique. Horizontal insertion, cephalad, 0.5 to 1.0 inches deep.
Moxa heating. 5 to 15 minutes.

4. Ru-kêng, *nipple line (Fig. 43)*

Location. Between the fifth and sixth ribs directly inferior to the nipple.
Indications. Mastitis and insufficiency of lactation.
Technique. Horizontal insertion in a cephalad, medial, or lateral direction to a depth of 0.5 to 1.5 inches.
Moxa heating. 5 to 20 minutes.

Table 3 cont.

LOCATION	NAME	COMMON INDICATIONS	SPECIFIC INDICATIONS
Leg and Foot	Chü-chüan Li-kou T'ai-ch'ung	Diseases of the liver *(Paralysis of lower extremity, diseases of abdomen and local area, urological disorders)*	Chü-chüan: Painful disorders of the knee and nocturnal emission Li-kou: Renal failure, impotence, nocturnal emission T'ai-ch'ung: Headache, dizziness, hypertension, mastitis, metrorrhagia
	Fu-liu T'ai-ch'i Yung-ch'üan	Diseases of the kidney	Fu-liu: Excessive perspiration, edema T'ai-ch'i: Painful disorders of the back and sole of foot Yung-ch'üan: Headache
Others	Pa-fêng Shang-pa-fêng Lin-hou		Pa-fêng and Shang-pa-fêng: Painful disorders of the foot and toes Lin-hou: Sciatica, paralysis of lower extremities

Points	General indications	Detailed indications
Yang-lin-ch'üan Tan-nang-hsüeh Chüeh-ku Ch'iu-hsü Tsu-lin-ch'i	Diseases of the eye, ear, chest, and gallbladder	Yang-lin-ch'üan: Painful disorders of the knee Tan-nang-hsüeh: Diseases of the gallbladder Chüeh-ku: Torticollis Ch'iu-hsü: Painful disorders of the ankle and rib cage Tsu-lin-ch'i: Painful disorders of the foot
Wei-chung Ch'êng-san K'un-lun Shu-ku Chih-yin	Diseases of the neck, eye, and nose; lumbago, sciatica	Wei-chung: Lumbago, painful disorders of the knee Ch'êng-san: Gastrocnemius spasm K'un-lun: Painful disorders of the ankle Shu-ku: Headache, dizziness Chih-yin: Malposition of fetus
Hsüeh-hai Yin-lin-ch'üan San-yin-chiao Shang-ch'iu Kung-sun Yin-pê	Disease of the stomach, intestines, and abdomen	Hsüeh-hai: Pruritus, menstrual irregularities Yin-lin-ch'üan: Abdominal distention, edema, urinary retention, painful disorders of the knee San-yin-chiao: Pruritus, diarrhea, diseases of the reproductive system, insomnia Shang-ch'iu: Painful disorders of the ankle Kung-sun: Diseases of the stomach and intestines Yin-pê: Menstrual irregularity

Paralysis of lower extremity, diseases of abdomen and local area, urological disorders

5. Chiu-wei, *xiphoid process (Figs. 43 and 44)*

   Location. 0.5 inches inferior to the xiphoid process.
   Indications. Psychoses, epilepsy, angina pectoris, emesis, and gastralgia.
   Technique. Diagonal insertion (30° angle), caudad, 1.5 to 2.0 inches deep.
   Moxa heating. 5 to 15 minutes.

6. Chung-kuan, *epigastrium (Figs. 43 and 44)*

   Location. At the epigastrium, 3.0 inches directly inferior to Chiu-wei (CA–5).
   Indications. Gastralgia, emesis, nausea, indigestion, gastroptosis, and abdominal distention.
   Technique. Perpendicular insertion 1.0 to 2.0 inches deep.
   Moxa heating. 10 to 20 minutes.

7. Ch'i-chung, *umbilicus (Fig. 44)*

   Location. At the umbilicus.
   Indications. Abdominal pain and diarrhea.
   Technique. No needle insertion is recommended.
   Moxa heating. 20 to 30 minutes.

8. Ch'i-hai, *upper hypogastrium (Fig. 44)*

   Do not use this point in pregnant women.
   Location. 1.5 inches directly inferior to the umbilicus.
   Indications. Nocturnal emission, impotence, menstrual cramps, menstrual irregularity, urinary retention, enuresis, diarrhea, and abdominal distention.
   Technique. Diagonal insertion, caudad, 0.8 to 2.0 inches deep. The bladder should be emptied before needle insertion.
   Moxa heating. 20 to 30 minutes.

9. Kuan-yüan, *mid-hypogastrium (Fig. 44)*

Do not use this point in pregnant women.
Location. 3.0 inches directly inferior to the umbilicus.
Indications. Nocturnal emission, impotence, menstrual cramps, menstrual irregularity, urinary retention, enuresis, diarrhea, and abdominal distention.
Technique. Diagonal insertion, caudad, 0.8 to 2.0 inches deep. The bladder should be emptied before needle insertion.
Moxa heating. 20 to 30 minutes.

10. Chung-chi, *lower hypogastrium (Fig. 44)*

Do not use this point in pregnant women.
Location. 4.0 inches directly inferior to the umbilicus.
Indications. Nocturnal emission, impotence, menstrual irregularity, excessive vaginal discharge, pelvic inflammatory disease,

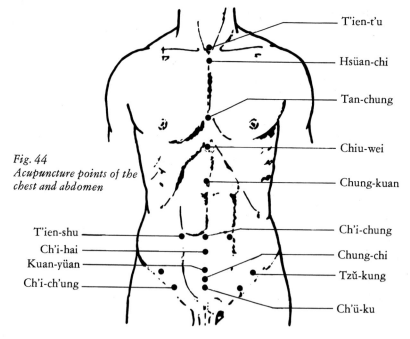

— T'ien-t'u

— Hsüan-chi

— Tan-chung

— Chiu-wei

— Chung-kuan

— Ch'i-chung

— Chung-chi

— Tzǔ-kung

— Ch'ü-ku

T'ien-shu —
Ch'i-hai —
Kuan-yüan —
Ch'i-ch'ung —

Fig. 44
Acupuncture points of the chest and abdomen

enuresis, urinary incontinence, and urinary retention.
Technique. Diagonal insertion, caudad, 0.8 to 2.0 inches deep.
The bladder should be emptied before needle insertion.
Moxa heating. 20 to 30 minutes.

11. Ch'ü-ku, *symphysis pubis (Fig. 44)*

Location. Immediately superior to the symphysis pubis.
Indications. Nocturnal emission, impotence, menstrual irregularity, excessive vaginal discharge, pelvic inflammatory disease, enuresis, urinary incontinence, and urinary retention.
Technique. Diagonal insertion, caudad, 0.8 to 2.0 inches deep. The bladder should be emptied prior to needle insertion.
Moxa heating. 20 to 30 minutes.

12. T'ien-shu, *paraumbilical (Fig. 44)*

Location. 2.0 inches lateral to the umbilicus.
Indications. Abdominal distention, diarrhea, menstrual disorders, constipation, and intestinal spasm.
Technique. Perpendicular insertion 0.7 to 1.2 inches deep.
Moxa heating. 10 to 20 minutes.

13. Ch'i-ch'ung, *lower inguinal (Fig. 44)*

Location. 2.0 inches lateral to the point Ch'ü-ku (CA–11).
Indications. Disorders of the male and female reproductive organs.
Technique. Perpendicular insertion 0.5 to 1.0 inches deep.
Moxa heating. 5 to 15 minutes.

14. Tzŭ-kung, *upper inguinal or uterus point (Fig 44)*

Location. 3.0 inches lateral to the point Chung-chi (CA–10).
Indications. Gynecological disorders.
Technique. Perpendicular insertion 1.5 to 2.0 inches deep.
Moxa heating. 10 to 20 minutes.

Table 4

SUMMARY OF ACUPUNCTURE POINTS OF THE CHEST AND ABDOMEN

LOCATION	NAME	COMMON INDICATIONS	SPECIFIC INDICATIONS
Chest	T'ien-t'u Tan-chung Hsüan-chi Ru-kêng	Diseases of the chest, including diseases of the upper respiratory system	T'ien-t'u: Diseases of the throat Tan-chung, Ru-kêng: Diseases of the breast
Upper Abdomen	Chiu-wei Chung-kuan	Diseases of upper abdomen, mainly diseases of the stomach	Chiu-wei: Mental disorders, epilepsy, chest pain Chung-kuan: Stomach and intestinal disorders
	Ch'i-chung T'ien-shu	Intestinal disorders	T'ien-shu: Menstrual disorders
Lower Abdomen	Ch'i-hai Kuan-yüan Chung-chi Ch'ü-ku	Urinary tract disorders and disorders of the reproductive system	Ch'i-hai, Kuan-yüan: Intestinal disorders
	Ch'i-ch'ung Tsŭ-kung	Disorders of the reproductive system	Tsŭ-kung: Gynecological disorders

POINTS OF THE BACK

1. Ta-ch'ui, *C7–T1* *(Fig.45)*

Location. In the midline between the seventh cervical vertebra (C7) and the first thoracic vertebra (T1).
Indications. Fever, malaria, schizophrenia, epilepsy, and asthma.
Technique. Perpendicular insertion 0.5 to 0.8 inches deep.
Moxa heating. 5 to 20 minutes.

2. T'ao-tao, *T1–T2 (Fig. 45)*

Location. In the midline between the first and second thoracic vertebrae.
Indications. Fever, malaria, and schizophrenia.
Technique. Perpendicular insertion to a depth of 0.5 to 0.8 inches.
Moxa heating. 5 to 20 minutes.

3. Ch'uan-hsi, *paravertebral C7 (Fig. 45)*

Location. 0.5 inches lateral to the seventh cervical vertebra.
Indications. Torticollis, asthma, and cough.
Technique. Perpendicular insertion 0.5 to 1.0 inches deep.
Moxa heating. 5 to 15 minutes.

4. Fêng-mên, *paravertebral T2–T3 (Fig. 45)*

Location. 1.5 inches lateral to the midline and at a level between the second and third thoracic vertebrae.
Indications. Influenza, pneumonia, bronchitis, asthma, pleurisy, pertussis, and upper backache.
Technique. Diagonal insertion, caudad, 0.3 to 0.5 inches deep.
Moxa heating. 5 to 15 minutes.

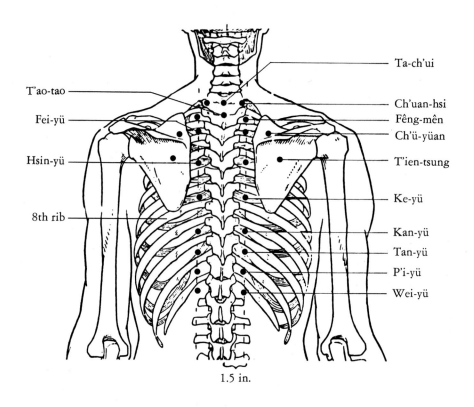

T'ao-tao

Fei-yü

Hsin-yü

8th rib

Ta-ch'ui

Ch'uan-hsi

Fêng-mên

Ch'ü-yüan

T'ien-tsung

Ke-yü

Kan-yü

Tan-yü

P'i-yü

Wei-yü

1.5 in.

Fig. 45
Acupuncture points of the back

5. Fei-yü, *paravertebral T3–T4 or lung point (Fig. 45)*

Location. 1.5 inches lateral to the midline and at a level between the third and fourth thoracic vertebrae.
Indications. Pneumonia, upper respiratory infections, asthma, pulmonary tuberculosis, pleurisy, cough, and upper backache.
Technique. Diagonal insertion, caudad, 0.3 to 0.5 inches deep.
Moxa heating. 5 to 15 minutes.

6. Hsin-yü, *paravertebral T5–T6 or heart point (Fig. 45)*

Location. 1.5 inches lateral to the midline and at a level between the fifth and sixth thoracic vertebrae.
Indications. Nervous breakdown, insomnia, palpitations, and schizophrenia.
Technique. Diagonal insertion, caudad, 0.3 to 0.5 inches deep.
Moxa heating. 5 to 15 minutes.

7. Ke-yü, *paravertebral T7–T8 or diaphragm point (Fig. 45)*

Location. 1.5 inches lateral to the midline and at a level between the seventh and eighth thoracic vertebrae.
Indications. Diaphragmodynia, upper backache, cough, asthma, and anemia.
Technique. Diagonal insertion, caudad, 0.3 to 0.5 inches deep.
Moxa heating. 5 to 15 minutes.

8. Ch'ü-yüan, *supraspinous fossa of scapula (Fig. 45)*

Location. Immediately superior to the medial border of the spine of the scapula in the supraspinous fossa.
Indications. Painful disorders of the scapula and shoulder.
Technique. Perpendicular insertion to a depth of 0.5 to 0.8 inches.
Moxa heating. 5 to 15 minutes.

9. T'ien-tsung, *infraspinous fossa of scapula (Fig. 45)*

Location. In the infraspinous fossa of the scapula at a point one-third the distance from the spine of the scapula to its inferior angle and midway between its medial and lateral borders.
Indications. Painful disorders of the shoulder, upper arm, and scapula.
Technique. Perpendicular insertion 0.5 to 1.5 inches deep.
Moxa heating. 5 to 15 minutes.

10. Kan-yü, *paravertebral T9–T10 or liver point (Fig. 45)*

Location. 1.5 inches lateral to the midline and at a level between the ninth and tenth thoracic vertebrae.
Indications. Hepatitis, backache, and diseases of the eye.
Technique. Diagonal insertion, caudad, 0.3 to 0.5 inches deep.
Moxa heating. 5 to 15 minutes.

11. Tan-yü, *paravertebral T10–T11 or gallbladder point (Fig. 45)*

Location. 1.5 inches lateral to the midline and at a level between the tenth and eleventh thoracic vertebrae.
Indications. Diseases of the gallbladder and bile ducts, hepatitis, and backache.
Technique. Diagonal insertion, caudad, to a depth of 0.3 to 0.5 inches.
Moxa heating. 5 to 15 minutes.

12. P'i-yü, *paravertebral T11–T12 or spleen point (Fig. 46)*

Location. 1.5 inches lateral to the midline and at a level between the eleventh and twelfth thoracic vertebrae.
Indications. Gastralgia, indigestion, anemia, and backache.
Technique. Diagonal insertion, caudad, 0.3 to 0.5 inches deep.
Moxa heating. 5 to 20 minutes.

13. Wei-yü, *paravertebral T12–L1 or stomach point (Figs. 45 and 46)*

Location. 1.5 inches lateral to the midline and at a level between the twelfth thoracic and the first lumbar vertebrae.
Indications. Gastralgia, indigestion, anorexia, and backache.
Technique. Diagonal insertion, caudad, 0.3 to 0.5 inches deep.
Moxa heating. 5 to 20 minutes.

14. Ming-mên, *L2–L3 (Fig. 46)*

Location. In the midline, between the second and third lumbar vertebrae.
Indications. Lumbar disorders, nocturnal emission, and impotence.
Technique. Perpendicular insertion 0.5 to 0.8 inches deep. The needle should be directed slightly cephalad.
Moxa heating. 5 to 20 minutes.

15. Shêng-yü, *paravertebral L2–L3 or kidney point (Fig. 46)*

Location. 1.5 inches lateral to the midline and at a level between the second and third lumbar vertebrae.
Indications. Lumbar disorders, renal infections, renal colic, nocturnal emission, impotence, menstrual disorders, and nervous breakdown.
Technique. Perpendicular insertion 0.5 to 1.2 inches deep.
Moxa heating. 5 to 20 minutes.

16. Chih-shih, *paravertebral L2–L3 (Fig. 46)*

Location. 3.0 inches lateral to the midline and at a level between the second and third lumbar vertebrae.
Indications. Lumbar disorders, renal infections, renal colic, nocturnal emission, and diseases of the reproductive system.
Technique. Either perpendicular insertion 0.3 to 0.5 inches deep

or horizontal insertion, cephalad or caudad, 1.0 to 2.0 inches deep.
Moxa heating. 5 to 20 minutes.

17. Yao-yang-kuan, *L4–L5 (Fig. 46)*

Location. In the midline, between the fourth and fifth lumbar vertebrae.
Indications. Lumbar backache.
Technique. Perpendicular insertion 0.5 to 1.2 inches deep.
Moxa heating. 5 to 20 minutes.

18. Ta-ch'ang-yü, *paravertebral L4–L5 or large intestine point (Fig. 46)*

Location. 1.5 inches lateral to the midline and at a level between the fourth and fifth lumbar vertebrae.
Indications. Lumbar and sacro-iliac strain, sciatica, painful disorders of the hip, and intestinal ailments.
Technique. Perpendicular insertion 0.7 to 1.3 inches deep.
Moxa heating. 5 to 20 minutes.

19. Shih-ch'i-ch'ui-hsia, *L5–S1 (Fig. 46)*

Location. In the midline between the fifth lumbar and first sacral vertebrae.
Indications. Sacro-iliac and hip pain.
Technique. Perpendicular insertion 1.0 to 2.5 inches deep.
Moxa heating. 5 to 20 minutes.

20. Shang-liao, *first sacral foramen (Fig. 46)*

Do not use this point in pregnant women.
Location. At the first sacral foramen, that is, 1.0 inches lateral to the midline of the sacrum and at a level between the first and second sacral vertebrae.

Indications. Urinary problems, menstrual irregularity, induction of labor, reproductive disorders, low backache, and sciatica.
Technique. Perpendicular insertion 1.0 to 2.0 inches deep.
Moxa heating. 5 to 20 minutes.

21. Ts'ŭ-liao, *second sacral foramen (Fig. 46)*

Do not use this point in pregnant women.
Location. At the second sacral foramen.
Indications. Similar to the indications for Shang-liao (B–20).
Technique. Same as technique for Shang-liao (B–20).
Moxa heating. 5 to 20 minutes.

22. Hsiao-ch'ang-yü, *paravertebral S1–S2 or small intestine point (Fig. 46)*

Location. 1.5 inches lateral to the midline and at a level between the first and second sacral vertebrae.
Indications. Low backache, hip pain, and intestinal disorders.
Technique. Perpendicular insertion 0.5 to 1.5 inches deep.
Moxa heating. 5 to 20 minutes.

23. P'ang-k'uang-yü, *paravertebral S2–S3 or bladder point (Fig. 46)*

Location. 1.5 inches lateral to the midline and at a level between the second and third sacral vertebrae.
Indications. Urinary disorders and low backache.
Technique. Perpendicular insertion 0.5 to 1.5 inches deep.
Moxa heating. 5 to 20 minutes.

24. Chih-pien, *paravertebral S4–S5 (Fig. 46)*

Location. 3.0 inches lateral to the midline and at a level between the fourth and fifth sacral vertebrae.
Indications. Sciatica, paralysis of lower extremity, gluteal pain,

anal disorders, and hemorrhoids.
Technique. Perpendicular insertion 1.0 to 2.0 inches deep.
Moxa heating. 5 to 20 minutes.

25. Ch'ang-ch'iang, *anal (Fig. 46)*

Location. In the midline, midpoint between the apex or tip of the coccyx and the anus.
Indications. Hemorrhoids and rectal prolapse.
Technique. With the patient bent over, perpendicular insertion, cephalad between the rectum and the coccyx, to a depth of 0.5 to 1.0 inches.
Moxa heating. 5 to 20 minutes.

26. Chiai-ch'uan, *paravertebral S1, S2, S3 (Fig. 46)*

Location. 2.0 inches lateral to the midline and at the levels of the first, second, and third sacral vertebrae, a total of three points on each side.
Indications. Cough and asthma.
Technique. Perpendicular insertion to a depth of 1.0 to 1.5 inches.

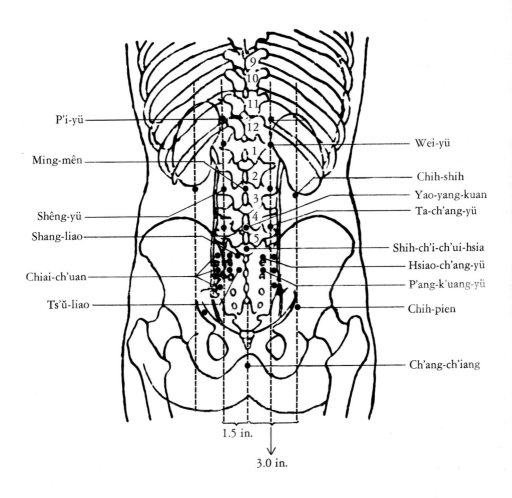

P'i-yü

Ming-mên

Shêng-yü

Shang-liao

Chiai-ch'uan

Ts'ŭ-liao

Wei-yü

Chih-shih

Yao-yang-kuan

Ta-ch'ang-yü

Shih-ch'i-ch'ui-hsia

Hsiao-ch'ang-yü

P'ang-k'uang-yü

Chih-pien

Ch'ang-ch'iang

1.5 in.

3.0 in.

Fig. 46
Acupuncture points of the lower back

Table 5

SUMMARY OF ACUPUNCTURE POINTS OF THE BACK

LOCATION	NAME	COMMON INDICATIONS	SPECIFIC INDICATIONS
Cervico-Thoracic	Ta-ch'ui T'ao-tao	Painful disorders of the vertebrae	Ta-ch'ui: Schizophrenia, asthma, fever, malaria T'ao-tao: Schizophrenia, fever, malaria
	Fêng-mên Fei-yü Ch'uan-hsi Hsin-yü Ke-yü	Local painful disorders — Diseases of heart and lung	Fêng-mên: Influenza Fei-yü: Diseases of the lung Hsin-yü: Diseases of the heart, mental disorders Ke-yü: Anemia, spasm of diaphragm Ch'uan-hsi: Asthma
Thoraco-Lumbar	Kan-yü Tan-yü P'i-yü Wêi-yü	Diseases of the liver, gall-bladder, spleen, stomach, and local soft tissue	Kan-yü: Diseases of the eye and liver Tan-yü: Diseases of the gallbladder P'i-yü and Wêi-yü: Indigestion, gastralgia
Lumbo-Sacral	Ming-mên Yao-yang-kuan Shih-ch'i-ch'ui-hsia	Diseases of the vertebrae	Ming-mên: Diseases of the male reproductive organ

Location	Points	Indications	Detailed indications
	Shêng-yü Chih-shih Ta-ch'ang-yü Hsiao-ch'ang-yü P'ang-k'uang-yü Shang-liao Ts'ü-liao Chih-pien	Diseases of the kidney, intestines, urinary tract, and reproductive organs Diseases of the local soft tissue	Shêng-yü, Chih-shih: Diseases of the urinary tract and reproductive organs Shang-liao, Ts'ü-liao: Diseases of the urinary tract and reproductive organs, sciatica Ta-ch'ang-yü, Hsiao-ch'ang-yü: Diseases of the intestines P'ang-k'uang-yü: Diseases of the urinary tract Chih-pien: Sciatica, paralysis of the lower extremity
Scapula	T'ien-tsung Ch'ü-yüan	Painful disorders of the shoulder	
Sacral	Chiai-ch'uan		Chiai-ch'uan: Cough, asthma
Anal	Ch'ang-ch'iang		Ch'ang-ch'iang: Hemorrhoids, rectal prolapse

POINTS OF THE EXTERNAL EAR

Acupuncture points of the external ear or auricle are, to a degree, unusual and unique in that they can be utilized for treatment of diseases of the entire body. They are noteworthy for achieving rapid alleviation of pain.

LOCATION OF ACUPUNCTURE POINTS

The auricle is pictured as a fetus in an inverted position in the uterus (see Figs. 47 and 48). With this in mind it is possible to ascribe to each organ of the human body a corresponding position in the auricle. Thus,

1. The lobule of the auricle is assigned to the face.
2. The antitragus is assigned to the head.
3. The antihelix is assigned to the spinal column.
4. The superior crus antihelicis is assigned to the lower extremities.
5. The inferior crus antihelicis is assigned to the buttocks.
6. The triangular fossa is assigned to the reproductive system.
7. The scaphoid fossa is assigned to the upper extremities.
8. The tragus is assigned to the nose, the throat, and the adrenals.
9. The incisura intertragica is assigned to the hormonal system and the scrotum.
10. The inferior concha is assigned to the thorax and its contents.
11. The superior concha is assigned to the abdomen and the following organs: kidney, urinary bladder, gallbladder, liver, and pancreas.
12. The crus helicis is assigned to the digestive system and the diaphragm.

SELECTION OF ACUPUNCTURE POINTS OF THE EXTERNAL EAR

As described in the preceding paragraph, each organ or structure of the body has a specific site on the auricle in which are located acupuncture points for treatment of its diseases or of symptoms arising from it. In addition, in accordance with medical theories, diseases of one organ may be due to afflictions of another organ. In such cases, the points for both organs are utilized. For example, practitioners of traditional Chinese medicine believe that diseases of the eye are related to disorders of the liver; therefore, acupuncture points specific for both organs are simultaneously used for treatment of these eye diseases. Furthermore, menstrual cramps are best treated by simultaneous stimulation of acupuncture points for the uterus as well as the hormonal system. For diseases of the internal organs, the specific points in both ears are used.

Technique. After the specific site of the auricle has been selected, the exact location for acupuncture is detected by:
1. Gently tapping the specific ear site with a needle to locate the most sensitive spot and thereby the acupuncture point.
2. Observing for physical changes such as discoloration (red or dark spots). In general, pain will be elicited from these discolored spots when pressure is applied to them.

Following identification of the point, a needle a half-inch long is inserted through the skin and into the cartilage but not through it. The patient should be warned of pain accompanying the needle insertion. The needle is then intermittently twirled for 15 to 30 minutes.

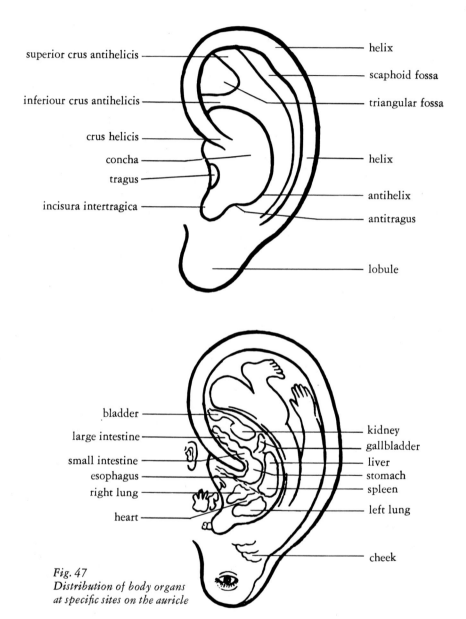

superior crus antihelicis

inferiour crus antihelicis

crus helicis

concha

tragus

incisura intertragica

helix

scaphoid fossa

triangular fossa

helix

antihelix

antitragus

lobule

bladder

large intestine

small intestine

esophagus

right lung

heart

kidney

gallbladder

liver

stomach

spleen

left lung

cheek

Fig. 47
Distribution of body organs
at specific sites on the auricle

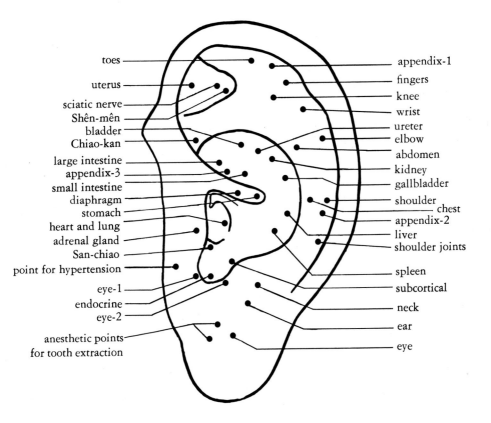

toes — appendix-1
uterus — fingers
sciatic nerve — knee
Shên-mên — wrist
bladder — ureter
Chiao-kan — elbow
large intestine — abdomen
appendix-3 — kidney
small intestine — gallbladder
diaphragm — shoulder
stomach — chest
heart and lung — appendix-2
adrenal gland — liver
San-chiao — shoulder joints
point for hypertension — spleen
eye-1 — subcortical
endocrine — neck
eye-2 — ear
anesthetic points — eye
for tooth extraction

Fig. 48
Distribution of ear acupuncture points

DISEASES AND SYMPTOMS
AMENABLE TO ACUPUNCTURE THERAPY

3   DISEASES AND SYMPTOMS
AMENABLE TO ACUPUNCTURE THERAPY

SELECTION OF POINTS FOR TREATMENT

In acupuncture therapy, treatment of a disease or symptom is accomplished by stimulation of a properly selected single acupuncture point or of a combination of several points. The number of main points or supplemental points to be used for a specific complaint varies, but in general is governed by the response to therapy. Certain diseases may improve dramatically by stimulation of just one or two of the main points specific for the disease, while others may require additional main points as well as supplemental points. In instituting treatment, it is customary to use the specific main points initially and, judging from the response, resort to supplemental points when necessary.

Acupuncture points are selected from one or a combination of the following categories of points:

1. Points situated in the proximity of the anatomical location of the disease or symptom. For example, the points for frontal headache, Yang-pê and Yin-t'ang; for temporal headache, T'ai-yang and Shuai-ku; and for goiter, Ch'i-yin.

2. Points situated at a distant site but which are held to exert a regulatory effect over specific diseased organs or the source of a symptom. These are exemplified by the specific points Lan-wei-hsüeh for appendicitis, Tan-nang-hsüeh and Nei-kuan for dis-

eases of the gallbladder and bile ducts, and Tsu-san-li, a main point for the amelioration of gastralgia and ileus.

3. Points selected for their efficacy in relieving specific symptoms. Noteworthy amongst these are the points Jen-chung and Shao-shang for syncope, Ta-ch'ui, Ch'ü-ch'ih and Ho-ku for fever, Nei-kuan and Tsu-san-li for nausea and emesis.

4. Pressure points which occur during the course of a disease. These points are usually found in the vicinity of the affected area, but they may also be located at a distant site, as in the case of the specific point for the treatment of appendicitis, Lan-wei-hsüeh, and also a main point for the treatment of diseases of the gallbladder and bile ducts, Tan-nang-hsüeh. Digital pressure on these pressure points will yield point tenderness prior to treatment of the condition.

5. Ear points. These points may be employed to complement the common acupuncture points.

Table 6

EXAMPLES OF COMBINATIONS OF LOCAL AND DISTANT ACUPUNCTURE POINTS IN THE TREATMENT OF DISEASES

DISEASE LOCATION		LOCAL ACUPUNCTURE POINTS	DISTANT ACUPUNCTURE POINTS
Head	Frontal	Yin-t'ang, Yang-pê	Ho-ku, Nei-t'ing
	Temporal	T'ai-yang, Shuai-ku	Chung-chu, Tsu-lin-ch'i
	Occipital	Fêng-ch'ih, T'ien-chu	Hou-ch'i, Shuai-ku
	Vertex	Pê-hui	T'ai-ch'ung
Eye		Ching-ming, Ch'êng-ch'i, Fêng-ch'ih	Ho-ku
Nose		Yin-t'ang, Yin-hsiang	Ho-ku
Mouth and teeth		Chia-ch'ê, Hsia-kuan, Ti-ts'ang	Ho-ku
Tongue		Lien-ch'üan,	Ho-ku
Throat		T'ien-yung	Ho-ku, Shao-shang
Trachea		T'ien-t'u	Lieh-ch'üeh
Lung		Fei-yü, Tan-chung, T'ien-t'u	Lieh-ch'üeh, Ch'ih-che
Heart		Hsin-yü, Tan-chung	Nei-kuan, Shên-mên, Chien-shih
Stomach		Wei-yü, Chung-kuan	Nei-kuan, Tsu-san-li
Liver		Kan-yü	T'ai-ch'ung
Gallbladder		Tan-yü	Tan-nang-hsüeh, Yang-lin-ch'üan
Intestines		Ta-ch'ang-yü, Hsiao-ch'ang-yü, T'ien-shu, Kuan-yüan	Shang-chü-hsü, Tsu-san-li
Kidney		Shêng-yü, Chih-shih	T'ai-ch'i
Bladder		Ts'ŭ-liao, Chung-chi	San-yin-chiao
Reproductive system		Chung-chi, Kuan-yüan, Tzŭ-kung	San-yin-chiao
Anus		Ch'ang-ch'iang, Chih-pien	Ch'êng-san
Upper extremity		Chien-yü, Ch'ü-ch'ih, Ho-ku	
Lower extremity		Huan-t'iao, Wei-chung, Yang-lin-ch'üan, Chüeh-ku	

Table 7

ACUPUNCTURE POINTS FOR TREATMENT
OF SPECIFIC SYMPTOMS

SYMPTOMS	ACUPUNCTURE POINTS (EXAMPLES)
Fever	Ta-ch'ui, Ch'ü-ch'ih, Ho-ku
Syncope	Jen-chung, Shih-hsüan
Shock	Tsu-san-li, Pê-hui, Kuan-yüan, Ch'i-chung
Excessive perspiration	Ho-ku, Fu-liu
Insomnia	Shên-mên, San-yin-chiao, T'ai-ch'i
Hoarseness	Ho-ku, Chien-shih, Fuh-t'u
Diarrhea	Shang-chü-hsü, T'ien-shu
Dysphagia	T'ien-t'u, Nei-kuan, Ho-ku, Fuh-t'u
Excessive salivation	Jen-chung, Chia-ch'ê, Ho-ku
Cough	T'ien-t'u, Lieh-ch'üeh
Heart palpitation	Nei-kuan, Hsi-mên
Chest pain	Tan-chung, Nei-kuan
Vomiting	Nei-kuan, Tsu-san-li
Dyspepsia	Tsu-san-li, Kung-sun
Dysarthria	Ya-mên, Lien-ch'üan, Ho-ku
Abdominal distention	T'ien-shu, Ch'i-hai, Nei-kuan, Tsu-san-li
Urinary retention	San-yin-chiao, Yin-lin-ch'üan
Incontinence of urine	Ch'ü-ku, San-yin-chiao
Impotence	Kuan-yüan, San-yin-chiao
Constipation	T'ien-shu, Chih-kou
Rectal prolapse	Ch'ang-ch'iang, Ch'êng-san
Gastrocnemius spasm	Ch'êng-san
Pruritus	Ch'ü-ch'ih, Hsüeh-hai
Chronic fatigue	Kuan-yüan, Tsu-san-li

LIST OF DISEASES AND SYMPTOMS

Enumerated here is a list of diseases and symptoms representative of ailments that are purported to respond well to acupuncture therapy. This list is selective and by no means complete. For each of the conditions mentioned, the common acupuncture points recommended for its treatment are listed. Also included are the ear points, whose usage, however, is optional.

SYNCOPE

Main points. Jen-chung (HN–18), Shao-shang (UE–23). Strong stimulation is recommended. The patient should be in Trendelenberg position.
Moxa heating. Pê-hui (HN–1).

MALARIA

Main points. Ta-ch'ui (B–1), T'ao-tao (B–2), Nei-kuan (UE–26), Chien-shih (UE–25).
Supplemental points. Ch'ü-ch'ih (UE–7), Tsu-san-li (LE–10), Yang-lin-ch'üan (LE–15).

Treatment should be instituted 2 to 3 hours before each episode of chills occurs. Strong stimulation for a brief period or intermittent twirling for 15 to 30 minutes is recommended.

UPPER RESPIRATORY INFECTIONS

Main points. Fêng-ch'ih (HN–25), Ho-ku (UE–12).
Supplemental points. Yin-hsiang (HN–17), T'ai-yang (HN–3), Fêng-mên (B–4), Ta-ch'ui (B–1).

ASTHMA

Main points. Ch'uan-hsi (B–3), T'ien-t'u (CA–1), Hsüan-chi (CA–2), Tan-chung (CA–3), Chiai-ch'uan (B–26).
Supplemental points. Ho-ku (UE–12), Tsu-san-li (LE–10).

Between the acute asthmatic episodes, any 2 to 4 of the main points along with the supplemental points may be used for treatment of the disease. Treatment is performed once daily and for a period of 7 to 10 days. For an acute attack, the main points Hsüan-chi and Tan-chung are used. Continuous twirling of the inserted needle for 2 to 5 minutes is recommended. If relief is not forthcoming, the main point Chiai-ch'uan is used in addition. This point is stimulated for 10 to 20 minutes.

Ear points. The point is located at the specific site for the lung.
Moxa heating. Ta-ch'ui (B–1), Fêng-mên (B–4), Fei-yü (B–5). Heating is to be applied only between asthmatic attacks.

COUGH

Main points. Fei-yü (B–5), T'ien-t'u (CA–1), Ch'ih-che (UE–20), Lieh-ch'üeh (UE–21), Ch'uan-hsi (B–3).

RHINITIS

Main points. Yin-t'ang (HN–6), Ho-ku (UE–12).
Supplemental points. Yin-hsiang (HN–17).

PHARYNGITIS, TONSILLITIS

Main points. T'ien-yung (HN–30), Ho-ku (UE–12).
Supplemental points. Shao-shang (UE–23), Ch'ü-ch'ih (UE–7).

Diseases and Symptoms

HYPERTENSION

Main points. Group 1: Ch'ü-ch'ih (UE–7), T'ai-ch'ung (LE–33). Group 2: Fêng-ch'ih (HN–25), Tsu-san-li (LE–10).
Supplemental points. T'ai-yang (HN–3), Yin-t'ang (HN–6), I-fêng (HN–28), Shên-mên (UE–30).

The two main groups may be alternately used. For symptomatic relief, the supplemental points are added: for temporal headache, T'ai-yang; for frontal headache, Yin-t'ang; for tinnitus, I-fêng; and for insomnia, Shên-mên.

Ear points. The point is located at the specific site for the heart.

NAUSEA AND EMESIS

Main points. Nei-kuan (UE–26).
Supplemental points. Tsu-san-li (LE–10), Chung-kuan (CA–6).

GASTRALGIA

Main points. Nei-kuan (UE–26), Tsu-san-li (LE–10).
Supplemental points. Chung-kuan (CA–6), Wei-yü (B–13).
Ear points. The point is located at the specific site for the stomach.
Moxa heating. Chung-kuan (CA–6), Tsu-san-li (LE–10). Heating is performed only between attacks of pain.

DYSPEPSIA

Main points. Chung-kuan (CA–6), T'ien-shu (CA–12), Ch'i-hai (CA–8), Tsu-san-li (LE–10).
Supplemental points. P'i-yü (B–12), Shêng-yü (B–15), Nei-kuan (UE–26), San-yin-chiao (LE–27).

Ear points. These are located at the specific sites for the stomach, intestines, and gallbladder.
Moxa heating. Any of the above points may be used.

For pediatric digestive disorders, the point Szŭ-fêng (UE–33) is used.

CONSTIPATION

Main points. Chih-kou (UE–14), T'ien-shu (CA–12).

DYSENTERY

Main points. Shang-chü-hsü (LE–12), T'ien-shu (CA–12).
Supplemental points. Nei-kuan (UE–26), Kuan-yüan (CA–9), Ch'ü-ch'ih (UE–7).

Intermittent twirling for 30 minutes is recommended for the point Shang-chü-hsü. The supplemental points Nei-kuan for emesis and Ch'ü-ch'ih for fever are added as necessary. Treatment is performed 1 to 3 times a day.

Ear points. These are located at the sites designated for the small and large intestines.
Moxa heating. Chung-kuan (CA–6), T'ien-shu (CA–12), Ch'i-chung (CA–7), Kuan-yüan (CA–9).

ILEUS (paralytic)

Main points. Tsu-san-li (LE–10), Nei-kuan (UE–26).
Ear points. The point is located at the specific site for the intestines.

HEPATITIS

Main points. Kan-yü (B–10), Tan-yü (B–11), Tsu-san-li (LE–10), T'ai-ch'ung (LE–33).
Supplemental points. Ta-ch'ui (B–1), I-ming (HN–29), Yang-lin-ch'üan (LE–15).

Diseases and Symptoms

The supplemental points Ta-ch'ui for fever, I-ming for depression, and Yang-lin-ch'üan for jaundice are added when necessary.

BILIARY COLIC

Main points. Tan-nang-hsüeh (LE–16), Nei-kuan (UE–26).
Ear points. These are located at the sites designated for the gallbladder and the liver.

APPENDICITIS

Main points. Lan-wei-hsüeh (LE–11), Ch'ü-ch'ih (UE–7), Nei-t'ing (LE–14).
Supplemental points. T'ien-shu (CA–12).

Intermittent twirling for 1 to 2 hours is recommended. Treatment is performed 2 to 3 times a day until the abdominal pain does not recur.

This treatment is not recommended when appendiceal rupture is suspected.

ENURESIS

Main points. Kuan-yüan (CA–9), San-yin-chiao (LE–27).
Supplemental points. Tsu-san-li (LE–10).
Ear points. Located at the specific site for the urinary tract.

IMPOTENCE

Main points. Kuan-yüan (CA–9), San-yin-chiao (LE–27).
Supplemental points. Shêng-yü (B–15), Tsu-san-li (LE–10).

RENAL COLIC

Main points. Shêng-yü (B–15), San-yin-chiao (LE–27).
Supplemental points. Chih-shih (B–16), T'ai-ch'i (LE–34).
Ear points. The point is located at the specific site for the urinary tract.

URINARY TRACT INFECTIONS

Main points. Ts'ŭ-liao (B–21), San-yin-chiao (LE–27), Chung-chi (CA–10), Ch'ü-ch'üan (LE–31).
Supplemental points. P'ang-k'uang-yü (B–23), Ch'ü-ch'ih (UE–7).
Ear points. The point is located at the site designated for the urinary tract.

HEADACHE

Frontal headache. The acupuncture points are Yin-t'ang (HN–6), Tsuan-tsu (HN–15), Ho-ku (UE–12), T'ai-ch'ung (LE–33).
Temporal headache. The acupuncture points are Fêng-ch'ih (HN–25), T'ai-yang (HN–3), Szŭ-tsu-k'ung (HN–16), Tsu-lin-ch'i (LE–19), Chung-chu (UE–17), Ho-ku (UE–12).
Occipital headache. The acupuncture points are Fêng-ch'ih (HN–25), T'ien-chu (HN–27), Hou-ch'i (UE–18), Shu-ku (LE–23), Ho-ku (UE–12).
Vertical headache. The acupuncture points are Pê-hui (HN–1), Fêng-ch'ih (HN–25), Ho-ku (UE–12), T'ai-ch'ung (LE–33).
Generalized headache. The acupuncture points are Fêng-ch'ih (HN–25), Ho-ku (UE–12), Pê-hui (HN–1), K'un-lun (LE–22).

TOOTHACHE

Main points. Ho-ku (UE–12).
Supplemental points. Chia-ch'ê (HN–9), Hsia-kuan (HN–8).

For toothache of the upper teeth, the supplemental point is Hsia-kuan; for the lower teeth, Chia-ch'ê.

Ear points. This point is located at the specific site for the cheek.

Diseases and Symptoms

TIC DOULOUREUX

Main points. Tsuan-tsu (HN–15), Szŭ-pê (HN–7), Hsia-kuan (HN–8), Chia-ch'êng-chiang (HN–21).

Supplemental points. Ho-ku (UE–12), Nei-t'ing (LE–14), T'ai-ch'ung (LE–33), Tsu-san-li (LE–10).

Opthalmic branch: The point Tsuan-tsu is used.
Maxillary branch: The point Szŭ-pê is used.
Mandibular branch: The points Hsia-kuan and Chia-ch'êng-chiang are used.

FACIAL NERVE PARALYSIS

Main points. I-fêng (HN–28), Szŭ-pê (HN–7), Yang-pê (HN–4), Ti-ts'ang (HN–19).

Supplemental points. Jen-chung (HN–18), Chia-ch'êng-chiang (HN–21), T'ai-yang (HN–3), Ho-ku (UE–12).

POLIOMYELITIS

Main points. Chien-yü (UE–2), Pi-nao (UE–8), Ch'ü-ch'ih (UE–7), and Ho-ku (UE–12) for paralysis of the upper extremities; Huan-t'iao (LE–1), Chih-pien (B–24), Yin-mên (LE–7), Fêng-shih (LE–6), Fu-t'u (LE–5), and Tsu-san-li (LE–10) for paralysis of the lower extremities.

Supplemental points. Chien-liao (UE–4) and Wai-kuan (UE–15) for the upper extremities; Yang-lin-ch'üan (LE–15), Chüeh-ku (LE–17), K'un-lun (LE–22), and T'ai-ch'i (LE–34) for the lower extremities.

For treatment of paralysis, three to six main points and two to four supplemental points are used for each treatment.

AMYOTROPHIA

For the upper extremities. Chien-yü (UE–2), Ch'ü-ch'ih (UE–7), Lieh-ch'üeh (UE–21), T'ai-yüan (UE–22), Ho-ku (UE–12).
For the lower extremities. Tsu-san-li (LE–10), Fêng-shih (LE–6), Huan-t'iao (LE–1), Yang-lin-ch'üan (LE–15), Chiai-ch'i (LE–13), T'ai-yüan (UE–22), Chüeh-ku (LE–17), Fu-t'u (LE–5).

The point Lieh-ch'üeh is specific for weakness of the wrist.

HEMIPLEGIA

Main points. Chien-yü (UE–2), Ch'ü-ch'ih (UE–7), Wai-kuan (UE–15), Ho-ku (UE–12), Huan-t'iao (LE–1), Fêng-shih (LE–6), Yang-lin-ch'üan (LE–15), Chüeh-ku (LE–17), Lien-ch'üan (HN–33).

Two to three of the main points from each afflicted extremity as well as the points Ch'ü-ch'ih and Yang-lin-ch'üan on the normal extremities are utilized in the treatment. The point Lien-ch'üan is specifically indicated for dysarthria.

EPILEPSY

Main points. Hsin-yü (B–6), Fei-yü (B–5), P'i-yü (B–12), Ta-ch'ui (B–1).
Supplemental points. Tsu-san-li (LE–10), Nei-kuan (UE–26).

INSOMNIA

Main points. Shên-mên (UE–30), San-yin-chiao (LE–27).
Supplemental points. Nei-kuan (UE–26), Yin-pê (LE–30), T'ai-ch'i (LE–34).

NEURASTHENIA

Main points. I-ming (HN–29), Shên-mên (UE–30), San-yin-chiao (LE–27).

Supplemental points. T'ai-yang (HN–3), Pê-hui (HN–1), Nei-kuan (UE–26), Chung-kuan (CA–6), T'ien-shu (CA–12), Kuan-yüan (CA–9), Ts'ŭ-liao (B–21), Tsu-san-li (LE–10).

HYSTERICAL BEHAVIOR

Main points. Jen-chung (HN–18), Nei-kuan (UE–26), Ho-ku (UE–12), T'ai-ch'i (LE–34), San-yin-chiao (LE–27).

This treatment is used in conjunction with orthodox psychiatric therapy.

SCHIZOPHRENIA

Main points. Group 1: Jen-chung (HN–18), Ho-ku (UE–12), T'ai-ch'ung (LE–33). Group 2: T'ai-yang (HN–3), Nei-kuan (UE–26), San-yin-chiao (LE–27).
Supplemental points. Ya-mên (HN–26), Ta-Ch'ui (B–1), T'ao-tao (B–2), T'ing-kung (HN–23), Ching-ming (HN–10).

Treatment is performed once or twice daily using the two groups of main points alternately. Best response is achieved by using all the points in the group simultaneously. Stimulation by twirling is maintained continuously or intermittently for one-half hour. A 26 gauge needle is used. If no response is noted in a week's time, supplemental points are added. As a rule, treatment is continued for a month on a daily basis, even after improvement is noted. Frequency of treatment can then be reduced to a weekly basis.

PELVIC INFLAMMATORY DISEASES, MENSTRUAL IRREGULARITIES AND CRAMPS

Main points. Kuan-yüan (CA–9), San-yin-chiao (LE–27).
Supplemental points. Ch'i-ch'ung (CA–13), Li-kou (LE–32), Hsüeh-hai (LE–25), Tsu-san-li (LE–10), Yin-lin-ch'üan (LE–26), P'i-yü (B–12), Kung-sun (LE–29).

Ch'i-ch'ung and Li-kou are specific supplemental points for pelvic inflammatory diseases; Hsüeh-hai, Tsu-san-li, and Yin-lin-ch'üan for menstrual irregularities; and Kung-sun for menstrual cramps.

Ear points. Located at the specific sites for the uterus, the ovary, and the hormonal system.

INDUCTION OF LABOR

Main points. Shang-liao (B–20), Ts'ŭ-liao (B–21), Ho-ku (UE–12), San-yin-chiao (LE–27).

DISEASES OF THE EYE

Main points. Ching-ming (HN–10), Fêng-ch'ih (HN–25), Ho-ku (UE–12).
Supplemental points. T'ai-yang (HN–3), Yang-pê (HN–4), Ch'iu-hou (HN–12), Ch'êng-ch'i (HN–11), Nei-kuan (UE–26), Tsu-san-li (LE–10).

The supplemental point T'ai-yang is added to the main points for the treatment of conjunctivitis and keratitis. Some blood should be produced from this point. For glaucoma, the supplemental points are Yang-pê and T'ai-yang; for optic neuritis and optic nerve atrophy, Ch'iu-hou and Ch'êng-ch'i. *The needle should not be twirled when it is inserted within the orbital rim.* Treatment is performed for 15 to 30 minutes daily for 10 to 15 days; it may then be resumed after a rest period of a week.

DEAFNESS AND MUTISM

Main points. Êrh-mên (HN–22), T'ing-kung (HN–23), T'ing-hui (HN–24), Ya-mên (HN–26), Lien-ch'üan (HN–33).
Supplemental points. Ho-ku (UE–12), Chung-chu (UE–17), Wai-kuan (UE–15).

Diseases and Symptoms

For deafness, the main points Êrh-mên, T'ing-kung, and T'ing-hui are used. When response is obtained, the points for mutism, Ya-mên and Lien-ch'üan, are added. In general, two or three of the main points, together with one of the supplemental points, are utilized. Performed once daily, the treatment is continued for 10 days. It is resumed after a rest period of 3 to 7 days. Intensive speech therapy is instituted as soon as the patient can hear.

TINNITUS

Main points. I-fêng (HN–28), I-ming (HN–29), T'ien-yu (HN–31), Fêng-ch'ih (HN–25).
Supplemental points. Chung-chu (UE–17), Wai-kuan (UE–15).

A combination of two main points and one supplemental point is used for each treatment.

MÉNIÈRE'S DISEASE

Main points. Fêng-ch'ih (HN–25), Nei-kuan (UE–26).
Supplemental points. I-fêng (HN–28), T'ing-kung (HN–23), Tsu-san-li (LE–10), Chung-kuan (CA–6).

The points Tsu-san-li and Chung-kuan are added to the main points when nausea is part of the symptomatology. If hearing is impaired, I-fêng and T'ing-kung should also be used.

GOITER

Main points. Ch'i-yin (HN–34), Ho-ku (UE–12).

LUMBAGO

Main points. Pressure points.
Supplemental points. Hou-ch'i (UE–18), Yin-mên (LE–7).

Ear points. Located at the specific site for the spinal column.
Moxa heating. Same as acupuncture points.

Best results are obtained by simultaneous application of acupuncture
and moxa heating.

SCIATICA

Main points. Huan-t'iao (LE–1), Yin-mên (LE–7), Yang-lin-ch'üan
(LE–15), pressure points.
Supplemental points. Shang-liao (B–20), Wei-chung (LE–20),
Ch'êng-san (LE–21).
Ear points. Located at the specific sites for the spinal column, the kid-
ney, and the point for the sciatic nerve.
Moxa heating. Same points as acupuncture points.

Best results are obtained by simultaneous application of acupuncture
and moxa heating.

PAINFUL DISORDERS, HIP

Main points. Huan-t'iao (LE–1), Chü-liao (LE–2).
Moxa heating. Same as acupuncture points.

Best results are obtained by simultaneous application of acupuncture
and moxa heating.

PAINFUL DISORDERS, KNEE

Main points. Nei-wai-ch'i-yen (LE–8), Liang-ch'iu (LE–9), Yang-
lin-ch'üan (LE–15), pressure points.
Supplemental points. Wei-chung (LE–20).
Moxa heating. Same as acupuncture points.

Best results are obtained by simultaneous application of acupuncture
and moxa heating.

PAINFUL DISORDERS, ANKLE

Main points. Chiai-ch'i (LE–13), Ch'iu-hsü (LE–18), pressure points.
Supplemental points. Chüeh-ku (LE–17).
Moxa heating. Same as acupuncture points.

Best results are obtained by simultaneous application of acupuncture and moxa heating.

PAINFUL DISORDERS, TOE

Main points. Pa-fêng (LE–37), Shang-pa-fêng (LE–38).
Moxa heating. Same as acupuncture points.

Best results are obtained by simultaneous application of acupuncture and moxa heating.

PAINFUL DISORDERS, HEEL AND SOLE OF FOOT

Main points. Pressure points.
Supplemental points. Ch'êng-san (LE–21), T'ai-ch'i (LE–34).
Moxa heating. Same as acupuncture points.

Best results are obtained by simultaneous application of acupuncture and moxa heating.

PAINFUL DISORDERS, SHOULDER

Main points. Chien-yü (UE–2), Chien-liao (UE–4), Nao-yü (UE–5), T'ien-tsung (B–9), Chien-nei-lin (UE–3), Chü-ku (UE–1), pressure points.
Supplemental points. Ch'ü-yüan (B–8), Pi-nao (UE–8), Yang-lin-ch'üan (LE–15).

For subscapular bursitis, the main points to be used are T'ien-tsung, Nao-yü, and Chien-nei-lin.

For subacromial bursitis, the main points recommended are Chien-yü, and Chien-liao.

For supraspinatus tendinitis, the main points are Chien-yü, and Chü-ku.

For tendinitis of the long head of the biceps muscle, pressure points are the main points.

In all of the above conditions, addition of the supplemental point, Yang-lin-ch'üan, is desirable.

Treatment is carried out every other day for a total of 7 to 10 treatments. If necessary, treatment may be resumed after a rest period of a week. Best results are obtained by simultaneous application of acupuncture and moxa heating.

Ear points. They are located at the specific site for the shoulder.
Moxa heating. Same as the acupuncture points.

PAINFUL DISORDERS, ELBOW

Main points. Ch'ü-ch'ih (UE–7), T'ien-ching (UE–13), Chou-liao (UE–10), pressure points.
Supplemental points. Yang-lin-ch'üan (LE–15).
Moxa heating. Same as the acupuncture points.

Best results are obtained by simultaneous application of acupuncture and moxa heating.

PAINFUL DISORDERS, WRIST

Main points. Yang-ch'ih (UE–16), Wai-kuan (UE–15), pressure points.
Supplemental points. Yang-ch'i (UE–11), T'ai-yüan (UE–22), Lieh-ch'üeh (UE–21).

For deQuervain's disease (stenosing tenosynovitis over the radial styloid), the main points are the pressure points. The supplemental points are Yang-ch'i, T'ai-yüan, and Lieh-ch'üeh.

For median nerve compression at the wrist, the main points are Ta-lin (UE–27), Shang-pa-hsieh (UE–32), and Nei-kuan (UE–26).

Moxa heating. Same as the acupuncture points.

PAINFUL DISORDERS, FINGER JOINTS

Main points. Pa-hsieh (UE–31), Shang-pa-hsieh (UE–32).

PAINFUL DISORDERS, MANDIBULAR JOINTS

Main points. Hsia-kuan (HN–8), Ho-ku (UE–12).

TORTICOLLIS

Main points. Pressure points in the neck and shoulders.
Supplemental points. Fêng-ch'ih (HN–25), Chüeh-ku (LE–17), Hou-ch'i (UE–18).

ISCHEMIA OF THE EXTREMITIES

Main points. Ch'ü-ch'ih (UE–7) and Shao-hai (UE–29) for upper extremities; Yang-lin-ch'üan (LE–15) and Yin-lin-ch'üan (LE–26) for the lower extremities.
Supplemental points. Shang-pa-hsieh (UE–32) for the upper extremities; Shang-pa-fêng (LE–38) for the lower extremities.
Moxa heating. Same as the acupuncture points.

This treatment is indicated for conditions such as intermittent claudication and Raynaud's disease.

NEURODERMATITIS

Main points. Ch'ü-ch'ih (UE–7), Hsüeh-hai (LE–25).
Supplemental points. Ho-ku (UE–12), San-yin-chiao (LE–27).
Ear points. Located at the specific sites for the lung, the liver, and the adrenal glands.
Moxa heating. Same as the acupuncture points.

133

ACUPUNCTURE-ANESTHESIA

4   ACUPUNCTURE-ANESTHESIA

Among the many contributions of contemporary medicine in the People's Republic of China, perhaps the most impressive achievement is the development of acupuncture-anesthesia, an accomplishment that truly reflects the successful integration of traditional Chinese medicine with Western science. Since its discovery in 1958, acupuncture-anesthesia has been safely utilized in more than 500,000 surgical operations with a success rate of approximately 90 percent. It varies in effectiveness mainly in the type of operation performed. Its advantages over conventional anesthesia in terms of tolerance, safety, economics, and simplicity are obvious. A patient "under" acupuncture-anesthesia is free of pain, but his other physiological functions remain unimpaired. He is conscious and mentally alert, allowing, in certain operations, the advantage of cooperation between surgeon and patient. Obviated are the postoperative complications and discomforts that attend conventional anesthesia.

Extensive clinical research in acupuncture-anesthesia has been conducted, and is continuing, in China and in some European countries, notably Soviet Russia. Suffice it to say that there is no scientific theory to date that can entirely explain all the physiological effects of acupuncture-anesthesia. There is, however, general agreement that different levels of the central nervous system are involved and that other systems, such as the humoral system, may also be participating factors.

Despite the resumption of communications between the United

States and the People's Republic of China, information pertaining to acupuncture-anesthesia unfortunately remains meager. The following comprises information that has been obtained mainly from current Chinese journals reporting on this all-important subject.

PRINCIPLES OF ACUPUNCTURE-ANESTHESIA

The technique of needle insertion for acupuncture-anesthesia is similar to the technique described for the treatment of disease. There are certain salient features, however, that are considered highly essential for the induction of acupuncture-anesthesia. First, it is imperative to obtain a strong sensory response (Te-ch'i) to acupuncture. This response must be maintained throughout the period of induction and anesthesia by continuous stimulation of the acupuncture points. Second, an induction or stimulation period of at least 20 to 30 minutes is advised in order to attain surgical anesthesia. Although continuous stimulation of the points may be performed by manual twirling combined with a rapid up-and-down movement of the needles, it is more practical to stimulate the points mechanically by attaching the needles to electrodes connected to a phasic battery power unit. The latter serves strictly as a labor-saving device and is especially advantageous in situations where multiple needles are inserted, in long surgical procedures, and in situations where operating space is limited and the acupuncture needles are, of necessity, inserted in the vicinity of the operative field.

Premedication may or may not be given, nor is it found essential for anesthesia. The patients are reassured and informed of what to expect. To compensate for possible respiratory embarrassment in chest operations such as thoracotomy and pulmonary resection, patients undergoing these operations are taught to "breathe with their abdominal muscles" for several days prior to surgery.

During the course of surgery, an analgesic, hypnotic, sedative, or local anesthetic may be added to supplement acupuncture-anesthesia when indicated. The analgesic effect of acupuncture-anesthesia does not end with cessation of the stimulation but persists for several hours.

When it does recede, it may again be induced by acupuncture. Except for occasional ecchymoses at the acupuncture sites, no post-anesthetic side effects have been reported.

SELECTION OF ACUPUNCTURE POINTS

Body points. Most acupuncture points for anesthesia are selected from the traditional acupuncture points described in Chapter 3. As a rule, this selection is based on knowing precisely which area or organ of the human anatomy is directly affected by stimulation of a specific acupuncture point. Thus, since pharyngitis, tonsillitis, and toothaches are relieved by stimulation of the point Ho-ku, it followed that this point would be used to induce anesthesia for surgery in the region of the pharynx and the mouth. Indeed, this was the point utilized for the first tonsillectomy performed under acupuncture-anesthesia. Similarly, Kung-sun and San-yin-chiao, two of several acupuncture points employed for the relief of abdominal disorders, are logically among those selected for acupuncture-anesthesia for abdominal operations. In a like manner, points for appendectomy (Lan-wei-hsüeh and T'ien-shu) and for thyroidectomy (San-yang-lo) were identified. The latter point, used in conjunction with the point I-fêng, also provides excellent anesthesia for chest operations such as thoracotomy and pneumonectomy.

Ear points. These points are very frequently utilized for acupuncture-anesthesia, either by themselves or in combination with acupuncture points in other locations. As in the treatment of diseases where each diseased organ or body area is treated by stimulating the acupuncture point located at its specific site at the external ear, anesthesia for the organ or area in question would be induced by the use of the appropriate ear point. Examples of combinations of ear points employed to achieve anesthesia for various surgical procedures are given in Table 8. These points are identified in Fig. 48. Several recent clinical studies to evaluate the efficacy of injecting various substances into the ear points to provide surgical anesthesia have reportedly yielded

promising results. Included were injections of small quantities (0.1 to
0.2 cc.) of extracts of Chinese herbs and Vitamin B_1 into the organ-
specific points in both ears.

Table 8

EXAMPLES OF EAR POINTS FOR
ACUPUNCTURE-ANESTHESIA

OPERATION	EAR POINTS*	BODY POINTS**
Eye operations	Eye-1, Eye-2	
Thyroidectomy	Neck	
Mastectomy	Chest, Subcortical	Nei-kuan, Ho-ku
Gastrectomy	Stomach, Large intestine, Small intestine, Spleen	Ke-yü, Wei-yü
Splenectomy	Spleen, San-chiao	Ke-yü, P'i-yü
Cholecystectomy	Spleen, Gallbladder	Ke-yü, Tan-yü
Nephro-ureterolithotomy	Kidney, Bladder, Subcortical	Shêng-yü, Wei-yü Tan-yü
Appendectomy	Appendix, Chiao-kan or Large and Small intestine	Lan-wei-hsüeh, Ta-ch'ang-yü
Gynecological operations	Uterus, Endocrine	

* These combinations of ear points are used with either of the following groups of main ear points: (1) Shên-mên, Lung; (2) Abdomen, Lung.
** These body points are frequently used in conjunction with the ear points.

Selection of Points

Nose points. Acupuncture points for every organ or area of the body are also found on the nose (Fig. 49). These points are mainly used for acupuncture-anesthesia. The following report from the People's Hospital, Tseng-chen County, Canton Province (1972), describes the effectiveness of selected nose points in providing acupuncture-anesthesia for various surgical operations (Table 9). The selected nose points utilized in this report were:

1. The lung point, located at the midpoint between the eyebrows.

2. The heart point, located at the midpoint between the medial canthus of the eyes.

3. The liver point, located 0.5 cm. directly below the heart point.

4. The supplemental point #1, located at the upper end of the alar fold of the nose.

5. The supplemental point #2, located between the tip and the alar of the nose.

6. The point Ts'ang-hsin-hsüeh, located midway between the nostrils, at the level of their upper margins and directly below the point for the reproductive organs.

7. The point Tsŭ-pao-hsüeh, located at the anterior nasal spine.
Acupuncture of these selected nose points was accomplished in the following manner: Only four needles were employed for all the points. The first needle was horizontally inserted in a cephalo-caudad direction, beginning slightly above the lung point, passing through the heart point, and terminating at the liver point, embracing all three of these points. The insertion was facilitated by depressing the nose. Also with the nose depressed, the second needle was horizontally inserted, passing from supplemental point #1 to supplemental point #2. In similar manner, a third needle was inserted for the contralateral supplemental points. For the insertion of the fourth needle, the tip of the nose was tilted upwards. The needle was then passed through the columella, beginning at the point Ts'ang-hsin-hsüeh and incorporating and ending at the point Tsŭ-pao-hsüeh.

Table 9

EFFICACY OF ACUPUNCTURE-ANESTHESIA WITH NOSE POINTS

OPERATION	TOTAL		EXCELLENT		GOOD	FAIR	FAILURE
	No. of cases	% success	No. of cases	%	No. of cases	No. of cases	No. of cases
Gastrectomy, gastroenterostomy, intestinal operations	180	99.4	131	72.7	25	23	1
Splenectomy	13	92.3	8	61.5	2	2	1
Cholecystectomy, common duct exploration	7	100.00			7		
Nephrectomy, ureterolithotomy, cystolithotomy, prostatectomy, cystorraphy, cystectomy	16	100.0	8	50.0	7	2	
Hysterectomy, Caesarean section, tubal ligation, oophorectomy	60	98.3	42	70.7	11	6	1
Appendectomy, exploratory laparotomy	26	100.0	9	34.6	13	4	
Thyroidectomy	21	100.0	13	61.9	7	1	

I. Excellent = Acupuncture-anesthesia alone was sufficient.
II. Good = Hypnotics, sedatives, or analgesics were added to supplement acupuncture-anesthesia.
III. Fair = Local anesthetic was added to I and II.
IV. Failure = Conventional anesthesia was needed for completion of operation.
V. % success = Includes excellent, good, and fair results.

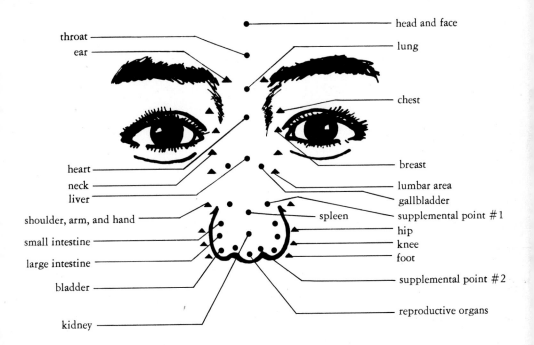

throat

ear

head and face

lung

chest

breast

heart

neck

liver

shoulder, arm, and hand

small intestine

large intestine

bladder

kidney

spleen

lumbar area

gallbladder

supplemental point #1

hip

knee

foot

supplemental point #2

reproductive organs

Fig. 49
Acupuncture points of the nose

In general, acupuncture-anesthesia for a particular surgical procedure is achieved by stimulation of not just only a single acupuncture point but a combination of several points. However, it has been observed in retrospect that during the early stages of the development of acupuncture-anesthesia, frequently more than the necessary number of points was employed to induce anesthesia for a specific operation. Through clinical experience, the trend has been to reduce the necessary number of points whenever feasible. Directly related to this effort is the recent observation that the stimulation of just one point, San-yang-lo, is sufficient to induce anesthesia for thyroidectomy and chest operations.

There is, reportedly, no absolute contraindication to the use of acupuncture-anesthesia. However, apprehensive patients are considered poor candidates for this type of anesthesia. Inadequate muscle relaxation and patient discomfort with traction on the viscera have been significant drawbacks in abdominal operations when acupuncture-anesthesia was used. In these operations, acupuncture-anesthesia is not recommended for patients who have thick abdominal musculature and when considerable visceral traction is anticipated, as could occur in the presence of extensive adhesions.

This form of anesthesia is considered most effective for surgical procedures of the head, neck, and chest. It is employed in infants as well as the aged and is ideally suited for patients of high surgical risk, due either to debilitation or serious concurrent diseases. Although much experimentation is still transpiring in this field, acupuncture-anesthesia is at present the anesthetic of choice in China, even though it is still regarded as an addition to, and not as a replacement for, conventional anesthesia.

BIBLIOGRAPHY

SOURCES

With the exception of the Preface and the Introduction, the information in this text was compiled and translated from the publications listed below.

Chên Chiu Chih Liao Hsüeh [*Treatment by Acupuncture and Moxibustion*]. Edited by School of Chinese Traditional Medicine, Shanghai, 1960.

針灸治療學 - 上海市中医學院編

Chên Chiu Chih Liao Shou Ts'e [*Handbook of Acupuncture and Moxibustion Treatment*]. Edited by Academy of Acupuncture, Shanghai, 1971.

針灸治療手冊 - 上海市針灸研究所編

Chên Chiu Lin Ch'uang Ch'ü Hsüeh T'u Chiai [*Diagrammatic Illustrations of Acupuncture and Moxibustion Points*]. Edited by School of Chinese Traditional Medicine, Peking, 1971.

針灸臨床取穴圖解 - 北京中医學院編

Chên Chiu Yü Hsüeh Hsüeh [*Locations of Acupuncture and Moxibustion Points*]. Edited by School of Chinese Traditional Medicine, Shanghai, 1960.

針灸腧穴學 - 上海市中医學院編

Chung I Tsa Chih [*Journal of Chinese Medicine*], no. 10, 1959.

中医杂志

Hsin I Hsüeh [*New Medicine*], no. 9, 1971. 新医學

Hsin I Hsüeh [*New Medicine*], no. 10, 1971.

Hsin I Hsüeh [*New Medicine*], no. 4, 1972.

Peking Review, Feb. 1972.

Bibliography

REFERENCES

The following list contains complete citations for works discussed in the Introduction.

Choain, J. La *"voie rationelle" (Tao) de la medicine chinoise*. Lille: Editions s.l.e.l., 1957.

Dimond, E. G. "Acupuncture Anesthesia, Western Medicine, and Chinese Traditional Medicine." *JAMA* 218 (1971): 1558–63.

Man, Pang L. and Calvin H. Chen. "Acupuncture 'Anesthesia'—A New Theory and Clinical Study." *Current Therapy Researches* 14 (no. 7, July 1972): 390–94.

Melzack, R. and P. D. Wall. "Pain Mechanism: A New Theory." *Science* 150 (1965): 971–81.

Peking Acupunctural Anesthesia Coordinating Group. "The Principle of Acupunctural Anesthesia." *Peking Review* 15 (nos. 7–8, 25 February 1972): 17–18.

Ramussen, T. and Wilder Penfield. "Further Studies of the Sensory and Motor Cerebral Cortex of Man." *Proceedings, Federation of Biological Sciences* 6 (1947): 452–60.

Tien, H. C. "Acupuncture Anesthesia: Neurogenic Interference Theory." *World Journal of Psychosynthesis* (1972): 36–41.

Toyama, Philip M. and Michimasa Nishizawa. "The Physiological Basis of Acupuncture Therapy." *North Carolina Medical Journal* 33 (no. 6, May 1972): 425–29.

Veith, Ilza. "Acupuncture Therapy—Past and Present—Verity or Delusion." *JAMA* 180 (May 1962): 478–84.

Veith, Ilza, tr. *Huang Ti Nei Ching Su Wen* [*The Yellow Emperor's Classic of Internal Medicine*]. Berkeley, Calif.: University of California Press, 1966.

148

INDEXES

INDEX OF
ACUPUNCTURE POINTS

HN designates points of the head and neck.
UE designates points of the upper extremity.
LE designates points of the lower extremity.
CA designates points of the chest and abdomen.
B designates points of the back.

INDEX OF DISEASES
AND SYMPTOMS

Index of Diseases and Symptoms

Date Due